AFTER YOU HEAR IT'S CANCER

AFTER YOU HEAR IT'S CANCER

A Guide to Navigating the Difficult Journey Ahead

John Leifer
with Lori Lindstrom Leifer, MD

ROWMAN & LITTLEFIELD
Lanham • Boulder • New York • London

Published by Rowman & Littlefield
A wholly owned subsidiary of The Rowman & Littlefield Publishing Group,
Inc.
4501 Forbes Boulevard, Suite 200, Lanham, Maryland 20706
www.rowman.com

Unit A, Whitacre Mews, 26-34 Stannary Street, London SE11 4AB

British Library Cataloguing in Publication Information Available

Library of Congress Cataloging-in-Publication Data

Leifer, John, 1957-
After you hear it's cancer : a guide to navigating the difficult journey ahead / John Leifer ; with Lori
Lindstrom Leifer.
pages cm
Includes bibliographical references and index.
ISBN 978-1-4422-4625-6 (cloth : alk. paper) -- ISBN 978-1-4422-4626-3 (electronic)
1. Cancer--Popular works. 2. Cancer--Patients--Popular works. 3. Cancer--Treatment--Popular
works. I. Leifer, Lori Lindstrom. II. Title.
RC263.L369 2015
616.99'4--dc23
2015000013

∞™ The paper used in this publication meets the minimum requirements of
American National Standard for Information Sciences Permanence of Paper
for Printed Library Materials, ANSI/NISO Z39.48-1992.

Printed in the United States of America

CONTENTS

PROLOGUE

A Life-Changing Experience

While many people revel in Christmas, my wife loves the sanctity of Easter. So it was no surprise Lori wanted to attend sunrise Easter services on March 31, 2013. The service was jubilant, and we spent the day feeling that all was right with the world.

When I finally crawled into bed around 11:00 p.m., I began to drift, though I wanted to stay awake until Lori finished her shower. A few minutes later, Lori quietly drew back the covers and slid into bed. I woke long enough to tell her I loved her and give her a short kiss.

Then I was out—until her sobs summoned me back to consciousness. "What's wrong? What's going on? What did I do?" I asked.

There was no response for what felt like an eternity. Then, in an uncharacteristically weak voice, Lori said, "I found something in the shower."

"What do you mean you found something in the shower?" I said anxiously.

"I found a lump. It is two centimeters. It's cancer."

Not only had Lori found a lump in her breast, but also, as an oncologist, she had determined its size and that it was malignant. I knew she was a great doctor, but I prayed there was room for error. Many times during our marriage, I hoped Lori was wrong, but never more than at this moment.

My wife, a radiation oncologist, would soon go from being a provider of care to a receiver of it. Lori and I would gain a new perspective about why the word *cancer*, rolling slowly and menacingly from our physicians' mouths, rattles us to the bone. It is a word we hope never to hear—certainly not in the context of our health or the health of a loved one.

> When you hear the word *cancer*, it's as if someone took the game of Life and tossed it in the air. All the pieces go flying. The pieces land on a new board. Everything has shifted. You don't know where to start.
>
> —Regina Brett[1]

As one patient said, "I thought I was going to die. I thought I was going to pass out. I was upset. I called my roommate and I was hysterical. I didn't know what to do. I was like blown away. It was a complete shock. To me, ovarian cancer is a death sentence."[2] Yet cancer is part of the human condition. It strikes approximately one-third of women and one-half of men at some point in their lives. In 2014, an estimated 1.66 million people received a diagnosis of cancer. They joined a pool of 13.7 million Americans already living with cancer, the vast majority of whom are fifty-five or older.[3]

Overall, newly diagnosed cancer patients will have a 68 percent chance of surviving for five years or more—a dramatic gain from forty years ago, when the survival rate was less than 50 percent. Even so, nearly 600,000 Americans will die from cancer this year, making cancer the second-leading cause of death in our country.[4]

If you're lucky, the journey will be a short divergence from life's path. For some, however, it will be a dramatic fork in the road to an unknown future. For all, it is a life-changing diagnosis.

A JOURNEY OF UNKNOWN DURATION AND DESTINATION

Imagine going on a trip without knowing the destination or method of transportation, with no map to guide you and no planned arrival time. Now imagine you are leaving tomorrow, and there is no time to pack. It is little wonder that cancer patients often feel overwhelmed, shut down, and are unable to participate in crucial decisions about their care. Our logical minds stop working just when we need to be thinking with absolute clarity about our next steps.

Karen Sepucha, a professor at Harvard Medical School and one of the leading authorities on how patients make crucial health care decisions, explained it to me this way:

> By the time people face cancer, they've usually faced other major issues in their life and made other difficult decisions. What I have found is that, sometimes, when they get into the medical community, they forget all of that. So people who have pretty advanced ways of taking care of their families and making good decisions all of sudden get to the doctor's office and lose all of the skills that allow them to question things, get other opinions—things that they would do in any other aspect of their life.[5]

It is a moment when time stands still, a moment laden with anxiety and uncertainty. A new journey is beginning, and it is one for which we are ill prepared. Just ask Bill E.

Bill E. is a retired school principal with a quick and beguiling smile. His easygoing nature does little to betray his unbending spirit. It is the kind of spirit needed to work with troubled kids, which was Bill's passion throughout a career spanning more than forty years.

As an African American growing up in rural Missouri in the 1950s, Bill faced plenty of challenges. In fact, Bill believed he was prepared for just about anything that life could throw at him—until he confronted cancer.

It was shortly after his retirement when Bill first noticed a lump in his neck. His primary care doctor sent him to a specialist—an ear, nose, and throat doctor—who gave Bill an antibiotic and scheduled a follow-up in three months.

When the lump was still present on reexamination, the ENT ordered a biopsy. Bill's life was about to come to a screeching halt. When the doctor told him he had cancer, Bill's first thought was, "You're kidding me. I just retired. I want to live this new life!"

"You are not really sure, are you?" he asked his doctor.

"Yes," came the unflinching response.[6]

As a patient with a head and neck cancer, Bill faced a very tough road ahead. "I teared up and said, 'This cannot be happening to me.' I had worked all of my life and tried to do the right thing. I pray to God. I go to church. So I'm asking myself if this can really be. I felt like I had no alternative but to die."[7]

Bill's journey through cancer had begun in earnest.

While no book can alleviate the emotional or physical challenges brought on by cancer, it can provide a roadmap to navigating the journey ahead—whether blessedly short or arduously long.

WHAT WE HOPE YOU'LL GAIN

There will be crucial junctures along your journey—times when you need to make decisions regarding your treatment. These decisions can have a dramatic impact on your final destination as well as on how taxing your trek will be. Our job is to heighten your awareness of those times when such decisions arise and empower you with tools and information to make informed and appropriate choices.

Our navigational guide comes complete with a topographical map of the terrain ahead, including what to expect before, during, and after treatment. As you will discover, health care can be highly fragmented in its delivery as well as variable in its depth, breadth, and quality of services. Such variability makes good navigation an essential survival skill.

Finally, we hope to prepare you for the emotional roller-coaster ride that you and your loved ones will likely experience.

Lori and I will judge our success by the degree to which we have helped you navigate a complex health care system, feel empowered to make astute decisions at difficult junctures, and manage the emotional turbulence along the way.

THE INDIVIDUALS JOINING US ON OUR JOURNEY

Before we begin, I want to introduce you to the patients and caregivers who, in addition to Lori, put aside their concerns about privacy to talk about their very intimate journey through cancer. They hope that, by sharing their journeys through cancer, it can somehow lighten your load.

- **Bill E.** You met Bill earlier in this chapter, a retired high school principal who was looking forward to enjoying a leisurely life and spending time with his children and grandchildren—that is, until cancer threw a wrench into his plans. Bill had to struggle through the hardships of a neck cancer, including chemotherapy and radiation.

- **Dana B.** Dana is a warm and inviting fifth-grade teacher. It is easy to understand why she is loved and appreciated by her students and colleagues. She is married and has two daughters, one in high school and one in college. Dana was diagnosed with stage 3A breast cancer and underwent bilateral mastectomies, chemotherapy, and radiation.

- **Darrell H.** Darrell is an associate pastor at one of the nation's leading churches. Though not a cancer survivor, Darrell cared for his wife, Patricia, for more than twenty years as she endured lymphoma and then leukemia. He offers a rare glimpse into the life of the surviving caregiver—one rich with insight and emotion.

- **Diane C.** Diane has the unusual distinction of being both a cancer survivor and a surviving caregiver. Diagnosed in 2007 with acute leukemia, Diane was given a 20 percent chance of survival. Thanks to a bone marrow transplant, she remains cancer free. As she was adapting to the challenges of survivorship, her husband, Rick, was diagnosed with metastatic melanoma.

- **Myra C.** Few people in America understand end-of-life issues better than Myra. As the cofounder of one of the nation's premier bioethics think tanks, Myra has been immersed in the challenges of hospice and palliative care for many years. She recently served on the Institute of Medicine's committee addressing palliative care in America. Myra was diagnosed three and a half years ago with a rare form of ovarian cancer.

- **Shelley W.** Shelley was only thirty-seven years old when she was diagnosed with stage 2B invasive ductal carcinoma of the breast. Her tumor was "triple negative" (its growth was not regulated by such hormones as estrogen), meaning that it was more aggressive and potentially treatment resistant. She underwent surgery, including the removal of twenty-one lymph nodes, accompanied by thirty-three radiation treatments. She is a model of resilience.

- **Stephen M.** Stephen is a college professor at a major Midwestern university. He is the author of four books. Stephen was sixty-five at the time of our interview, and he asserted that, as a master's class athlete, he had enjoyed near-perfect health—until he was diagnosed with early-stage prostate cancer.
- **Mary E.** Mary is Lori's nurse. After thirteen years in oncologic nursing, she has a firm handle on the challenges faced by cancer patients. That knowledge proved invaluable when she was diagnosed with breast cancer and found that she carried a genetic mutation known as BRCA.
- **Alta F.** Alta worked for the federal government for more than forty years, with thirty-six years spent with the U.S. Postal Service. Alta is a survivor. During her seventy-four years, she's battled three separate cancers: non-Hodgkin's lymphoma, breast cancer, and now a second bout with lymphoma. She credits her faith in God and strong support from family and friends for her resilience.
- **Ali H.** Ali worked in the food and beverage business for much of his life. Just as he was on the cusp of accepting a major position with a new company, he was diagnosed with a head and neck cancer. His treatment was incredibly arduous, but he made it through.

We are grateful to each of our interviewees for sharing their powerful and enlightening stories. As you will discover, the common theme that runs through each of these stories is the power of hope—even when hope is a difficult thing to muster.

I

Diagnosis and Treatment Planning

I

A DEFINITIVE DIAGNOSIS

Setting the Stage for Treatment

Despite the overwhelming fatigue she felt, Lori did not sleep a second after discovering a lump in her breast during a shower on Easter evening. She tried to find ways to distract herself—catching up on e-mail, reading her Bible, praying, and crying a lot.

In the early hours of dawn, we crawled out of bed and had our customary cup of coffee before laying out a plan for the day. Our world, once so safe and tidy, was changing at a frightening pace. And despite our collective experience in health care, we felt completely unprepared for the fog of uncertainty that now engulfed us.

The first call was to one of Lori's colleagues, a radiologist whose specialty was breast imaging. Not wanting to be intrusive, Lori forced herself to wait until eight o'clock before contacting the department of radiology at St. Joseph Medical Center. She would soon be on her way to work—facing a day packed with patients and struggling to keep a lid on her growing anxiety.

"Good morning, Mary. This is Dr. Lindstrom. May I please speak with Dr. K.?"

There was a pause as Lori listened intently to the reply, then hope seemed to wash from her face. With a faded voice, she responded, "I see. Well, please tell him that I called, and it is important."

Fortunately, Lori did not have to wait very long to hear from Dr. K.

"I've found a lump in my breast, and I need you to biopsy it as soon as possible," she told him when he returned her call.

Dr. K. did not hesitate. "It's my day off, but you can meet me at the hospital at one o'clock."

"Thank you so much. That's incredibly kind of you," she said before hanging up the phone. Turning to me, Lori said, "He'll do whatever is necessary—including an immediate biopsy—to determine what's going on."

If there was a shred of self-pity, Lori discarded it with abandon. She knew that immersing herself in patient care would make the hours pass by faster.

Lori's journey began with a quick trip to the mammography unit. The technologist tried her best to reassure Lori that the lump was likely benign, but she knew better. After the images were completed, the technologist had to agree with her. "Yes, it does look malignant."

"Even though I had already known," Lori said, "my heart still sank into my stomach as I felt a wave of nausea when the mammogram confirmed my suspicions."

Patience has never been one of my virtues, and that day was no exception. Though the process was flawlessly smooth, it felt like an eternity before a tech summoned me to an exam room, where Lori and I would hear Dr. K.'s findings.

He confirmed the mass seen on the mammogram had characteristic malignant features. He could feel the mass easily. "The imaging studies confirm what you thought. You appear to have a two-centimeter mass in the upper outer quadrant of your breast. It needs to be biopsied. We can do it right now, if you're ready."

It was standard operating procedure and exactly what Lori would have ordered.

The confirmation was both disheartening and strangely comforting. Not only had Lori been right, but she had also precisely estimated the size of the tumor.

"Yes, of course. Let's get it done," Lori responded.

Dr. K. asked if I wanted to observe, and I said, "Absolutely."

The procedure began with a series of injections into Lori's breast. While she lay stoically on her back, I winced with imaginary pain. Once the anesthetic had taken effect, Dr. K. prepared to insert a large bore needle into the core of Lori's tumor. He used a sonogram to guide the needle precisely to its target. This translates into a higher probability of properly sampling the tumor rather than the surrounding breast tissue while also minimizing the discomfort experienced by Lori. It was a procedure Dr. K. had performed innumerable times, making him highly proficient.

The images on the sonogram were astonishingly clear—in fact, too clear for my faint-at-the-sight-of-blood constitution. It looked like a Black & Decker drill was being repeatedly thrust deeply into Lori's breast. My wife never betrayed any discomfort.

The biopsy took only about twenty minutes, and then the tissue samples were on their way to a pathology lab. There, a pathologist would expose the cells to various chemical stains, examine them under a microscope, and render a definitive diagnosis.

When Lori's tissue samples arrived in her lab for analysis, Dr. V. blinked in disbelief as the name of her friend and colleague came into sharp focus.

The next day, the results were back. What Lori had felt in her breast on Easter night was definitively cancer.

People learn of their potential cancer diagnoses in a variety of ways. It is usually not a singular event but a process that unfolds from suspicion to a definitive diagnosis. It may begin during self-examination, a routine screening procedure, a doctor's visit, or during an unscheduled visit to the ER. Something is amiss; it may be cancer; more testing will be required for a confirmatory diagnosis. Even so, the alarm bells are already sounding.

For Dana B., a fifth-grade teacher with two nearly grown daughters, the alarm bells gradually intensified in volume, not reaching full crescendo for more than two years. In 2011, Dana had just stopped taking birth control pills, when she noticed something wrong with her breast:

> When I stopped taking birth control pills, I felt an almost immediate change in my breast, which I thought was because of the hormone changes. There was just a hardened sensation in my breast, so when I went for my mammogram, I pointed this out. They compared it to last year's mammogram and said it looked normal.
>
> I didn't balk. I thought that mammograms were the most accurate diagnostic test you could do for breast cancer. Still, I felt and saw some physical changes, which I brought back up with my primary care doctor, who said, "Maybe we should do an ultrasound." I

asked her if that was really necessary right now and if we could wait until my next mammogram, and she indicated that it would be okay to wait until my next mammogram.

A year later, my doctor felt some increased density in my breast, but when I went back for my mammogram, I was told it looked normal. They did observe, however, that there was some thickening that they did not feel on the other side, so they recommended that I have an ultrasound. After that, they said I needed a biopsy.

I consulted with a radiologist at St. Joseph Medical Center. He looked over all of the mammograms and at the ultrasound and said, "I don't see anything, but the physical changes in your breast concern me, and therefore let's do a biopsy."

So we did that on Friday. On Monday, I got a call at school from the nurse navigator [a dedicated resource for helping patients manage their care] saying that the radiologist wanted to see me, which is scary because you know what is coming. My husband picked me up from work and we went in. That is when the radiologist told me I had lobular carcinoma, which is hard to see on ultrasound and mammograms.

I was just numb but listened to what he had to say . . . and waited for the next part of the plan. I think that the scariest part is just waiting for all of the pieces to come together.[1]

If, like Dana, you are undergoing evaluation for a potential diagnosis of cancer, then you are approaching one of the first signposts on your journey. Your challenge at this point is to understand how the tests or procedures ordered by your doctors will aid in the diagnosis and staging of your disease.

THE FIVE CATEGORIES OF CANCER

Cancer is not a single disease but a loose collection of diseases with widely varying symptoms, treatments, and prognoses. Though they number in the hundreds, every type of adult cancer falls into one of five groups based on its origin within tissue and blood in our bodies. The following are the five major categories of cancer.

Carcinoma

This cancer forms in the epithelial tissue that covers or lines surfaces of organs, glands, or body structures. Cancer of the stomach lining, for example, is a carcinoma. Many carcinomas affect organs or glands that are involved with secretion, such as breasts that produce milk. Carcinomas account for 80 to 90 percent of all cancer cases.

Sarcoma

This malignant tumor grows from connective tissues, such as cartilage, fat, muscle, tendons, and bones. The most common sarcoma, a tumor on the bone, usually occurs in young adults. Examples of sarcoma include osteosarcoma (bone) and chondrosarcoma (cartilage).

Lymphoma

This cancer originates in the nodes or glands of the lymph system, which filters white blood cells and body fluids, or in such organs as the brain and breast. Lymphomas fall into two categories: Hodgkin's lymphoma and non-Hodgkin's lymphoma.

Leukemia

This is a blood cancer that originates in the bone marrow (white or red blood cells or platelets) and eventually spills into the bloodstream.

Myeloma

This cancer grows in the plasma cells of bone marrow. In some cases, the myeloma cells collect in one bone and form a single tumor, called a plasmacytoma. If the myeloma cells collect in many bones and form many bone tumors, it becomes multiple myeloma.

Some of these cancers manifest in subtle ways, and patients often initially dismiss their symptoms, as was the case with Diane C.

Diane proudly states that she is rarely sick and almost never misses a day of work. Yet in 2007, she found herself fighting an unremitting cold.

As the days wore on, her fatigue increased to the point that she sought treatment at an urgent care center. There, she received an antibiotic. Two rounds of antibiotics later, she was no better. It was time to go to her doctor:

> When I called my doctor, she told me that I needed to come in so we could figure out what was going on. She did a blood test and followed up by phone a few days later. My doctor asked that I come into the office and told me to bring my husband. She wouldn't tell me why. When we went in, she said that I had a type of blood disease and that I needed to see a hematologist/oncologist.
>
> They told me that the oncologist could not see me for a week. I called the office back, and they got me in to see another doctor the next day. I was so sick by then that Rick, my husband, went with me to the appointment.
>
> The oncologist told me that I had acute myeloid leukemia. I had no idea. I had a ringing in my ears . . . and I was exhausted but had assumed it was nothing.[2]

WHEN CANCER IS SUSPECTED

If your doctor suspects cancer, as was the case with Dana and Diane, he or she will rely on testing to confirm the hypothesis. The appropriate tests can help physicians:

- determine whether a growth is benign or cancerous,
- identify the type of cancer present,
- assign a stage to the cancer, and
- assign a grade to the cancer.

The more you know about your disease, the better you will be able to participate in your care and understand what to expect and what to question.

If it feels like you have been thrust into a foreign land, trying to converse in a language that is spoken with great fluency by your physicians but unfamiliar to you, relax. Until you become more comfortable with the nomenclature spoken by physicians, ask your doctor (or his or her nurse) for a translation into plain English.

THE FIVE TYPES OF TESTING

There are five tests commonly used to diagnose and describe the precise clinical attributes of your cancer. Often doctors deploy multiple tests to ensure there is optimal information for staging and treatment planning. Some of these tests are noninvasive and pose no potential threat to the health of the patient. Other tests are quite invasive and can have some degree of risk.

Physical Exams

Just as Dr. K. began his diagnostic process with a physical examination of Lori, your doctor will likely conduct a thorough physical examination to reveal any readily detectable signs of disease.

Laboratory Tests

Doctors use these tests to examine blood, urine, and other fluids to determine if there are deviations from the normal ranges of key components, such as white blood cells or the presence of certain proteins associated with various tumors, known as *tumor markers*, for example, CA-125 for ovarian cancer. These tests can also help monitor a patient's response to chemotherapy and other treatment modalities.

Lab tests are relatively noninvasive (such as simply drawing a blood sample) and involve little direct risk to the patient. The American Association for Clinical Chemistry sponsors a guide to the vast majority of laboratory tests at http://www.labtestsonline.org.

Diagnostic Imaging

Imaging techniques, such as X-rays, sonograms, MRI scans, CT scans, and PET scans, provide relatively noninvasive methods of gathering important information. Each modality offers a dramatically different perspective on a tumor. Whereas MRI and CT provide richly detailed images and thus a great depth of diagnostic information about a tumor, a PET scan provides a functional image designed to reveal whether the tumor activity has spread to other areas of the body.

There are risks associated with certain modalities, particularly when they involve repeated doses of radiation. Multiple CT scans, for instance, can expose patients to a cumulative dose of radiation that carries its own risk. There are also significant costs associated with the majority of these tests. The Radiologic Society of North America (RSNA) and the American College of Radiology offer detailed explanations at www.radiologyinfo.org.

Biopsies and Subsequent Pathology Findings

These tests are the "gold standard" for making a definitive diagnosis of cancer. They require the direct sampling of tissue. Doctors obtain samples by surgery, scope, or a hollow needle.

Some biopsies take place at the time of surgery and involve a technique known as "frozen sampling." Frozen sections provide a surgeon with valuable preliminary information about how he or she should proceed with a given operation.

Other biopsies can be done through a scope inserted into the throat, lung, esophagus, stomach, or colon. Some growths can be biopsied directly, such as those found in the skin, cervix, or prostate.

Because of their invasive nature, biopsies can involve significant risk, pain, and cost. It is important that you speak with your physician and understand these factors before consenting to any biopsy.

Genetic Testing

There are three different but related ways in which genetic testing can be used during the diagnostic and treatment planning phases of your journey: (1) A physician or genetic counselor may take a family history to identify any apparent predisposition toward cancer in the family. (2) Your doctor may have your blood, saliva, or other biological sample analyzed for the presence of certain genetic mutations. (3) An analysis of the genetic nature of your tumor may be ordered by one of your physicians to help determine treatment options and the potential for recurrence.

Whether it is a diagnostic imaging study, biopsy, or genetic test, your doctor(s) will determine what is needed to render the best care. For many types of tumors, they may use all five test modalities. Ideally, the testing should yield useful information on the type and stage of cancer you have.

WHEN FOUR OUT OF FIVE TESTS PROVED POSITIVE

Four out of five tests helped doctors confirm a diagnosis of cancer in the case of Steven M., a sixty-five-year-old political scientist, professor in the School of Public Affairs, and director of a social science research institute at a major midwestern university. He is the author of four books. Most importantly, he has been remarkably healthy: "I had basically had no health issues ever, which made the cancer a bit of a shock." He explains,

> A couple of weeks before my annual physical, I had what felt like a bout of prostatitis, though I've never had prostatitis. A couple of warm baths seemed to take care of it. I mentioned this to my family doctor during my annual physical, so in addition to a digital rectal exam, he ordered a PSA test.
>
> He had felt something abnormal during the physical exam, and the PSA was elevated (I believe it was 4.9). So he recommended that I see a urologist. The urologist repeated the exam and PSA, and the findings were the same. At that point, he recommended a biopsy. I talked to my doctor, and he said, "Let's just wait." So I scheduled another visit with my urologist several months later.
>
> I did some reading about all of this . . . including a white paper on prostate disease from Johns Hopkins. I continued to consult with my family doctor, who thought it made sense to go ahead and have the biopsy. By then, it was the holidays, and he said there was no big rush. So I scheduled my biopsy for early January.
>
> The prostate biopsy came back with a Gleason score of 3+3 (an indication of the presence of early-stage cancer cells). There were twelve cores. In three to four of the cores, about half of the tissues sampled had cancer cells present.[3]

CANCER ISN'T A TRUE-OR-FALSE QUESTION

You might think it is simple to determine whether a tumor is cancerous, but not all cases are as straightforward as those we have read about so far. The difficulty comes in the labeling and definition of cancerous versus potentially precancerous conditions. Some patients have cancerous cells that are totally self-contained or in situ. A common example of this condition is ductal cell carcinoma in situ (DCIS).

What is at stake here is more than mere semantics. As diagnostic imaging has become increasingly powerful, the ability to diagnose precancerous conditions and relatively indolent (slow-growing) cancers has expanded dramatically. According to a *New York Times* article, "Once doctors and patients are aware a lesion exists, they typically feel compelled to biopsy, treat, and remove it."[4]

If your diagnosis falls into this gray area, it is all the more important that you understand as much about your disease as possible to ensure that you ultimately receive the appropriate level of treatment.

SOMETIMES A DIAGNOSIS PROVES DIFFICULT

Sometimes it is difficult for doctors to diagnose cancer because its presentation is highly unusual. Such was the case with Patricia H., whose husband, Darrell, recounts her story:

> Our daughter was born in 1990. About a year later, Patricia said to me, "You know, I've got an awful lot of cold sores in my mouth." I told her to go see the doctor. The doctor, instead of saying "Here's some mouthwash that will take care of it," said, "We need to do some blood tests." He came back and told us that her counts were low and she should see a specialist.
>
> The specialists bandied back and forth for almost two years between lymphoma and lupus or some other type of autoimmune condition. There was a lot of uncertainty. At the same time, our daughter, Meghan, was not developing speech and was playing with toys in an odd, atypical manner. In November 1993, we had back-to-back days when one day we took Meghan to Shawnee Mission Medical Center, and they confirmed a diagnosis of autism; the next day we got the official confirmation of lymphoma for Patricia.

When the doctors finally settled on a diagnosis of lymphoma, they told us that it was a very unusual presentation of lymphoma because it was not in the lymph glands but rather in the bone marrow. They explained that Patricia's counts were low because the lymphoma cells were aggressive and were displacing bone marrow cells.[5]

Determining that Patricia had cancer was the beginning of a journey that would span more than two decades as her doctors went through the steps of first understanding and then treating her condition.

IDENTIFYING THE TYPE OF CANCER

Job 1 is to identify the type of suspected cancer. The cell type, coupled with the location of the primary tumor, defines the specific type of cancer. Hence, a patient can have an adenocarcinoma of the breast or a non-small cell cancer of the lung. Cell type can be a crucial indicator of the aggressiveness of the tumor. A patient with a small, basal cell cancer of the skin may have little reason for concern. However, a patient with a small melanoma of the skin may face a very different fate.

Cancer can also be described by its location, as well as by using one of five terms defining how far it has traveled from its source:

- **In situ:** Abnormal cells are present only in the layer of cells in which they developed [it is noninvasive and therefore has no immediate potential to spread]
- **Localized:** Cancer is limited to the organ in which it began, without evidence of spread
- **Regional:** Cancer has spread beyond the primary site to nearby lymph nodes or tissues and organs
- **Distant:** Cancer has spread from the primary site to distant tissues or organs or to distant lymph nodes
- **Unknown:** There is not enough information to determine the stage[6]

Lori had an invasive cancer, which is normally well defined and thus easier to remove. However, the sample also contained an element of lobular cancer, which tends to be more diffuse in the breast and is notorious for hiding on imaging studies.

The next step is to stage the cancer.

THE STAGE OF CANCER

The most important piece of information you need to know about your cancer is its *stage*. Stage is the dominant factor that determines both treatment and prognosis. The stage describes the extent or severity of a cancer. The stage can change as additional information about the patient's condition is revealed or as a result of the progression of the disease.

A number of methods are used for staging, with TNM staging being most common. It categorizes cancer based on the size and extent (reach) of the primary tumor (T); whether the cancer cells have spread to nearby (regional) lymph nodes (N); and whether metastasis (M), or spread of the cancer to other parts of the body, has occurred.

Each of the TNM characteristics contributes to an overall staging on a scale from 0 to 4, with letters used to more precisely define substages. Stage 0 defines a non-invasive or precancerous condition, such as DCIS. Stages 1 to 3 indicate progressively more extensive disease that begins locally and spreads regionally. Stage 4 describes cancer that has spread to distant sites in the body.

The pathologist classified Lori's tumor as stage 2A, primarily based on its size being equal to or greater than two centimeters. Fortunately, there was no evidence of cancer in her lymph nodes, which would have increased her stage and the likelihood of recurrence.

Cancers are not only staged but also graded.

THE GRADE OF CANCER

Pathologists assign a numerical *grade* to most cancers depending on the appearance of the cancer cells under a microscope. They consider cells that closely resemble normal tissue as "well differentiated." These tumors generally tend to grow and spread at a slower rate than tumors that are "undifferentiated" or "poorly differentiated," which have more abnormal-looking cells and can lack normal tissue structures.

Most tumors are assigned a grade from 1 to 3. Grade 1 is a slower-growing tumor, while grade 3 is an undifferentiated, high-grade tumor that can grow and spread quickly. However, different systems are used for different types of tumors.

The Gleason score is a unique grading system used only in prostate cancer. The overall score is determined by adding together the two most common patterns of abnormal cells seen in patients' prostate biopsies using a scale from 1 to 5. The score ranges from 2 (1+1) to 10 (5+5). A score of 2 indicates cells that deviate only slightly from normal and suggests less likelihood of the cancer spreading, whereas a Gleason score of 10 would describe a highly undifferentiated and dangerous tumor. Steven's tumor scored a 3+3, which indicated an intermediate form of cancer.

Whatever the methodology, the intent is always to indicate the relative aggressiveness of the tumor and probability of spread.

HOW TO PARTICIPATE IN THE DIAGNOSTIC PHASE OF YOUR JOURNEY

One of the best ways to feel empowered during this early phase of your journey is by asking questions. Yet many patients are hesitant to do so, either believing that their physician knows what is best for them or that they simply should not appear to be questioning the physician's judgment. Some patients have had bad experiences with physicians who recoiled when asked to explain or justify a particular recommendation. Other patients struggle even to formulate which questions to ask.

It is essential that you be comfortable asking questions of your doctor and that you receive appropriate and satisfactory responses. Here are some of the questions you may wish to consider:

- What information do you hope to glean from test results?
- What are the clinical indications or reasons for recommending the test?
- How might the test results influence your recommended treatment options?
- What, if any, dangers or complications can arise from the test?
- How urgent is the need for the test?
- What is the cost/benefit of the test?
- How much discomfort or pain will I experience?
- What form will the results take?

You probably aren't going to grill your physician before a simple blood test, but you may want to do extensive research before consenting to a biopsy, costly imaging study, or other invasive tests.

Once you are properly informed, you will be in a better position to evaluate your comfort level with the physician's recommendations. Be sure to ask when and how you will receive the results of your tests. You want to be sure he or she knows you want information as soon as it becomes available.

The diagnostic phase represents a pivotal time in your journey. It is a time when you need to be exquisitely aware. Though every impulse may be urging you to shut down and numb out, the more clearly you can think, the more you can participate in impending decisions about your care. You need to fight with all of your might to overcome the raw fear gripping you.

PEER-TO-PEER REVIEWS

You may not be the only one asking your physician to explain his or her reason for ordering particular tests. Insurance companies are scrutinizing such decisions with increasing frequency—particularly relative to diagnostic imaging studies, which can costs thousands of dollars.

Your insurance company may ask your doctor to participate in a peer-to-peer review, during which he or she explains the rationale for a test to a physician employed by the insurance company. Based on the merits of your doctor's argument, the insurance company can opt to approve or deny the claim. If it is denied, either your physician must forgo the tests or you must pay out of pocket for them.

SOMEONE BY YOUR SIDE

We know from research how important it is for patients to have a strong support system of family and friends to help them get through cancer treatment. A trusted caregiver is a bit like your personal Sherpa—they help to lighten your load. Your caregiver can be a spouse, significant other, adult child, close friend, or relative. The caregiver's role needs to remain malleable, but in the early stage, it often includes a number of basic functions. Ideally, your caregiver will be present at your doctor appointments. You will be receiving information at breakneck speed—too quickly to assimilate it by yourself. That is why your caregiver needs to listen, record, and be able to recount what took place during these visits.

There is often a gap between what patients believe they heard and what their physicians assert they said. You may well be operating in crisis mode and have trouble retaining information. In these instances, the caregiver can capture the key elements of each discussion.

You will have information overload during this part of your journey. Physicians' use of arcane language further complicates understanding your diagnosis and making astute decisions. Research demonstrates that patients often fail to understand what they are being told. Thus, they may consent to procedures without appreciating the ramifications of such interventions.

Your caregiver can help you avoid this problem by speaking up and asking your physician to translate what he or she has said into lay terms. The caregiver can provide an important point of view as you work through the risks, limitations, costs, and other factors associated with the testing and treatment your doctor recommends.

Finally, your caregiver can provide emotional support. Do not underestimate the toll that cancer will take on you and your family. Though there are emotional challenges you must bear alone, an empathetic caregiver can be a godsend during stressful times. It's important to keep in mind, though, that your caregiver will not be immune to the forces that rattle your psyche. In fact, they will likely mirror your emotional struggles.

Shelley W., a thirty-nine-year-old mother and busy executive diagnosed with invasive breast carcinoma, described her husband's role: "He was very level headed about the approach to the process and treatment and served as my 'data guy,' memorizing statistics and keeping the notes from appointments. He was scared about what might happen to me but armed with as much knowledge as we could get to make good decisions along the way."[7]

When asked about her diagnosis, Shelley said, "Stage 2B invasive ductal carcinoma. My tumor size category is T2 and lymph node status or 'N level' is N1. I also have a subtype of cancer called 'triple negative breast cancer.' I am also negative for the BRCA gene mutation."[8]

Obviously, both she and her husband had done an excellent job of arming themselves with the facts. Every cancer patient and his or her caregiver learn these lessons. As Lori's caregiver, I would come to understand this all too well.

2

HOW PROGNOSIS INFLUENCES YOUR TREATMENT

Based on the results of her diagnostic imaging tests and biopsy, Lori appeared to have early-stage breast cancer. The tumor appeared well defined, which meant she was a likely candidate for a lumpectomy. It was clear that we needed a surgical opinion. Lori chose Dr. M., a colleague with whom she shared a great many cases. Lori was impressed with his calm, steady, and reassuring demeanor and his knowledge of breast cancer. He took time to explain each patient's diagnosis and how it translated into a probable prognosis.

After a perfunctory knock on the exam room door, Dr. M. paused briefly before opening it slowly. He greeted us with a warm smile and expression of genuine concern. Before beginning his examination of Lori, Dr. M. spent time talking to us about the situation—gathering information and, just as importantly, building rapport.

Once he had completed the physical exam, he pulled the pathology report from Lori's chart and began to discuss the biopsy results with us. Dr. M. spoke slowly and simply—not for Lori's benefit but to ensure that I, as a non-physician, understood everything he said. Only then was he ready to share his recommendations:

> Lori, based upon the tumor size and characteristics, I am recommending a lumpectomy followed by radiation. As you know, the data clearly demonstrates this approach is equally efficacious to mastectomy in preventing recurrence in early-stage breast cancer patients.

Furthermore, your recovery will be far shorter, the pain and discomfort minimal, and there will be no need for reconstruction.

Lori nodded but remained concerned: "But Dr. M., my tumor is at least two centimeters and appears to contain a lobular component. Are you confident that this is the right approach? Maybe I should even be considering bilateral mastectomies."

"You can certainly opt for a mastectomy, and some women do have bilateral mastectomies in the hope of reducing any probability of recurrence. I'm relatively certain that your insurance would cover the more extensive surgery. If, however, you choose to have a lumpectomy, on the small chance that we discover more advanced disease, then we can always perform a second surgery."

An almost imperceptible smile crossed Lori's lips; it was the momentary flicker of recognition. "I never understood before why stage 1 breast cancer patients opted for mastectomies when the data support minimal surgery. Now that I'm facing the same decision, I get it. I don't want to worry about whether or not you got all of the cancer. I want it out. I'd rather go through more surgery than risk having missed something."

Lori looked at Dr. M., then to me, and finally down at the floor. "I know I am reacting emotionally instead of with my head. I guess I need a day or two to think about it."

"Of course, take all the time you need, and call me once you've reached a decision. I know that whatever decision you make, it will be the right one for you."

AN INESCAPABLE REALITY

Once your test results are in hand, your physician formulates a diagnosis. In an instant, the threat of cancer is transformed from an abstract concept to a concrete reality: There is an invader within your body.

Shelley W. described her experience:

> By the time we got to that meeting with the surgeon, we knew it was cancer from the language in the preliminary reports. So we weren't surprised, but I did cry when she said I'd need a mastectomy, I think because it made it a little more real. Instead of being something that

happens to other people, it was happening to me. I don't recall feeling particularly scared or sad, but a little mad about what it meant for the future.[1]

Patients and caregivers often describe their diagnosis as a twofold process: First they stoically absorb the facts on an intellectual level, and only later are they bowled over by the emotional reaction to their situation. It is an extraordinarily difficult and confusing time, as was related by a forty-year-old leukemia patient who recalled being so overwhelmed by the conversations with different specialists that nothing seemed real for some time.[2]

Diane C. said that she was "in complete denial. I thought, 'OK, I am ill, but I will get through it.' But my husband understood just how serious it was." What neither Diane nor her husband, Rick, could have anticipated was that Rick would fall victim to an equally devastating form of cancer.

The inescapable reality of cancer eventually breaks through our defenses.

UNDERSTANDING ONE'S PROGNOSIS

While a diagnosis confirms the reality of cancer, a prognosis reveals what may lie ahead. It represents your physician's best estimate of the projected course of your disease over time. As such, it defines the anticipated end point of your journey.

Far from being an exact science, prognosticating is an art that blends the objective facts about your condition with statistical evidence of how other comparable patients have fared. A dose of your physician's intuition can be added liberally to this mix before yielding a final prognosis.

The two greatest determinants of your prognosis are the nature of the tumor as determined by location, size, stage, and grade and your performance status. Of the two, most experts agree, "The single most important predictive factor in cancer is Performance Status ('functional ability,' 'functional status'): a measure of how much a patient can do for themselves, their activity and energy level."[3] In simpler terms, your journey through cancer is influenced by the characteristics of your specific disease combined with your underlying health and vitality.

Your physician may use a scale to measure your performance status and functional ability. The two scales most frequently utilized by oncologists are the Eastern Cooperative Oncology Group (ECOG) scale and the Karnofsky index.

There are additional factors that can influence prognosis, as was the case with Myra C. when there was an unexpected rupture of her tumor at the time of surgery:

> I knew that I had a mass—having become aware of it around Thanksgiving. I wanted to get through the holidays and take care of year-end stuff, so I planned to call the doctor on January 16. I actually marked the calendar.
>
> On the night of January 15, we were out to dinner with good friends. When we started to leave, I almost collapsed from a horrific pain. We got home, and I wasn't fine. I couldn't sleep and kept pacing the floor. I kept wondering if I could wait until my doctor's office opened. I did. When I got in to see him, the first thing he said was, "We need to get you to the ER. It will be faster than if I just admit you."
>
> At first, they thought I might have a blockage in my bladder, but they ruled that out. They thought it might be a cancer. I told them I was not going to have surgery that night. They said, "Yes, you are going to do this tonight." The mass had shifted and was pressing against my spine.
>
> The hospital did not have a gynecologic oncologist on staff, so they began to call around to see who they could find to operate. A physician came in whom I had never met.
>
> In the surgery, they found a mass about the size of a child's football. It had attached to the wall of my endometrium [uterus]. As they were trying to remove it, it ruptured. My endometrium was flooded with cancer cells.[4]

Myra had several factors in her favor, including excellent functional status, tremendous tenacity, and a long list of medical experts ready to come to her aid. However, she also had a high-grade tumor that had ruptured during surgery.

THE FOUNDATION OF TREATMENT PLANNING

Diagnosis and prognosis combine to form the very foundation of treatment planning. For patients who wish to participate in treatment decisions, an "accurate prediction and disclosure of diagnosis and prognosis are essential for both treatment and personal decision-making."[5] This information appears to be beneficial in other ways, too.

Research studies have consistently illuminated the beneficial aspects of information sharing. For instance, when eighty-three cancer patients were interviewed by researchers in one study, they considered information sharing to serve three main functions: enabling them to actively participate in their treatment, reducing anxiety, and enabling them to prepare and plan for the future.[6] Conversely, a "lack of information, explanation, and support has been cited as the greatest cause of anxiety and stress in cancer patients."[7]

Unfortunately, several major impediments stand in the way of full and accurate disclosure, including the following:

- Physicians appear to have a bias toward unwarranted optimism when delivering difficult news to patients: "Research has shown that physicians are systematically overly optimistic in formulating survival estimates and even more optimistic when they disclose prognostic information to patients and/or their families."[8] As healers, it is understandable that they want to deliver hope. However, false hope can be as or more deleterious than withholding information.

- Patients and their families have a difficult time understanding the objective reality of their conditions: "Patients and families do not always translate metastatic disease to mean incurable disease, which is usually, but not always, the actual meaning of the situation. Furthermore, the word *respond* (as in 'a certain percentage of cancer patients will respond to treatment') is often misinterpreted by patients and families as *cured* ('a certain percentage will be cured')."[9]

Sometimes, the answers patients seek are not apparent to even their physicians, as was the case with Bill E. "They couldn't tell me what I wanted to know: Where did it come from, and what are the chances of me getting rid of it? I wanted to know, even if it was bad news. So I'm worrying, 'Is this in my brain?'"[10]

HOW MUCH DO YOU REALLY WANT TO KNOW?

Now might be a good time to ask yourself how much information do you want your physician to disclose about your condition? The truth about one's diagnosis and prognosis can be either uplifting or usher in a harsh, new reality. For some patients, a future, once meticulously planned, can change with the utterance of a few words by their doctors.

Despite the risks of reducing hope and injuring our psyches, the majority of patients want to know the truth, albeit to varying degrees of completeness. Here is a sampling from the hundreds of research studies examining this issue:

- "Our findings suggest that most people do want honest information, even if the news is bad. We found that 27 of 27 enrolled patients initially reported wanting to know all the available information about their cancer, prognosis, treatment benefits, and treatment side effects."[11]
- "Four relatively early studies reported that almost all patients (96–98%) wanted to be told whether their illness was cancer. Ten studies showed that many patients (57–95%) wished to receive all the information available, both good and bad. Four studies reported that most patients wanted to know about their chance of a cure (91–97%) and how effective the treatment of their cancer was (79–98%). However, four studies suggested that a lower percentage of patients (27–61%) wished to discuss their life expectancy."[12]
- "Most oncology patients also want to know their prognosis and have rated prognostic information as the most important element of communication—more important than diagnostic disclosure or treatment information."[13]
- "Younger patients, female patients and more highly educated patients consistently desired to receive as much detailed information as possible and to receive emotional support. Younger and more

highly educated patients also wanted to participate in decisions regarding their treatment."[14]

Regardless of what the research tells us, the bottom line is that there is no right or wrong when it comes to seeking or avoiding information about your prognosis. Despite what many research studies reveal, there are still many patients who are quite content to remain comfortably uninformed about certain stark realities. They may claim that they want to know everything but may not be ready to receive the information when they do.[15]

Dana B. knew what information she did and did not want to receive from her physician:

> I *did* want to know how the staging happened, but I *did not* want to know my likelihood of five-year survival. Different people handle things in different ways. For me, if someone told me that I had a 30 percent chance of living for five years, my hope just went down, whereas if I go into it blindly—not knowing the percentage—then I can make it in my mind whatever I want it to be. I'm naturally pessimistic, so to maintain optimism, I need to not go there with the numbers.[16]

So once again, before you ask your physician for more information about your diagnosis and prognosis, ask yourself, "How much do I want to know about my disease?" The Medscape website suggests cancer patients consider how they might respond to the following questions from their physician:

- Many patients want to know the prognosis. Is this true for you?
- Some people might not want to know how the cancer will affect survival but wouldn't mind someone telling their families. What do you prefer?
- What are you expecting to happen?
- How specific do you want me to be?[17]

RELIGIOUS, ETHNIC, AND CULTURAL VARIATIONS IN NORMS REGARDING DISCLOSURE OF INFORMATION

Your religious beliefs, as well as ethnic and or cultural background, can have a powerful impact on the manner in which you and your physician manage your disease. It is important that your doctor be aware of and sensitive to your needs in this regard.

PHYSICIANS PROTECTING US FROM THE TRUTH

If the majority of patients want to hear the truth about their conditions, why do physicians fail to deliver it? Lori and I believe that the primary reason dates back to one of the core tenets of medicine. Since the days of Hippocrates, one of medicine's guiding principles has been the admonition to physicians to *do no harm*. This ideal was codified more than a century ago in the American Medical Association's code of ethics, which reminded physicians of their duty to "avoid all things which have a tendency to discourage the patient and depress his spirits," for this constituted harm. [18]

This attitude toward patients did not change until recently. Until the 1970s, doctors could still get away with claiming they withheld information for the patient's own good. [19] In a recent survey, such paternalism was still evident: "Several doctors explained that they would only provide detailed information about prognosis if a patient specifically asked for it, because they were not convinced that providing time frames or statistical information was in a patient's best interest." [20]

There are other reasons physicians shield patients from information—including the simple fact that physicians, like the majority of mankind, would prefer to avoid difficult and painful discussions. Who can blame physicians, particularly when you realize that they have received little to no training on how to manage such conversations with their patients?

A LITTLE FINESSE GOES A LONG WAY

"What can make a huge difference . . . is how and how often doctors discuss options with patients and describe the potential of continued treatment." Two leading cancer experts quoted in a *New York Times* article suggest that practitioners master "ask, tell, ask," which consists of asking patients what they want to know about their prognosis, telling them what they want to know, and then asking, "What do you now understand about your situation?"[21]

Today, protecting patients from the truth has been replaced with a new guiding principle: The art of healing is a collaborative process that occurs between patient and physician. They are, in essence, partners in the care transaction. As one physician noted in a *New York Times* editorial, "[Patients] have the right to direct their own care, and to do so they must be fully informed. As doctors, we no longer 'care for' as much as 'care with' our patients through their illnesses."[22]

HOW OFTEN PHYSICIANS WITHHOLD INFORMATION

Despite the changing mores of health care, doctors commonly fail to ask what information patients want. In fact, the evidence consistently shows that doctors are hesitant to divulge prognostic information.[23]

The problem is particularly acute with patients facing terminal illness. Numerous studies have explored the levels of physician disclosure and have come to the following conclusions:

- "U.S. physicians do not disclose prognosis at least half the time and feel unprepared to have these discussions."[24]
- "Even if terminally ill patients with cancer requested survival estimates, doctors would provide such estimates only 37% of the time, often an overestimate; and a recent meta-analysis showed that cancer physicians consistently overestimated prognosis by at least 30%."[25]
- "Strikingly, physicians give the least honest figures to those with the worst prognoses (and perhaps most in need of information to make decisions). In one study, physicians who had referred patients to hospice reported that if the patient asked about progno-

sis, they would provide an honest estimate only 37% of the time. Most of the time, physicians would provide no estimate or a conscious overestimate."[26]

- "A study of 140 patients with metastatic cancer in the Netherlands found only 39% were told their prognosis by their oncologist. Similarly, an Australian study of patients with breast cancer or melanoma found only 27% were given a prognosis during their initial oncology consultation, while 57% desired this information."[27]

All of us want modern medicine to rescue us from a potentially devastating disease. The truth is that some of us will be rescued and some of us won't, but the vast majority of cancer patients will be blessed with many happy and productive years following their diagnoses.

HOW ACCURATE ARE PHYSICIANS IN TELLING THE FUTURE?

The short answer is *not very accurate*: "Clinical prediction of survival has been found to be erroneous (defined as more than double or less than half of actual survival) 30% of the time in expert hands. Two thirds of errors are based on over-optimism and one third on over-pessimism."[28]

Physicians seem to have an optimistic bias regarding patients' prognoses, as previously discussed. Once again, the patients least likely to receive an accurate appraisal of their future are those with the most advanced disease.

Studies evaluating the accuracy of doctors' survival predictions in patients with terminal cancer have been undertaken for more than thirty years. Most have looked at the difference between predicted survival and actual survival after the patient was referred to a palliative care service (noncurative clinical interventions designed to reduce pain and improve quality of life) or admitted to a hospice. A recent systematic review of eight such studies, four involving more than 1,500 predictions, showed the following results:

- Predictions were more than twice as likely to be overly optimistic (median predicted survival of six weeks versus median actual survival of four weeks).
- Predictions were correct to within a week in only 25 percent of cases.
- Predictions were off by more than a month in over 25 percent of cases.
- Despite the inaccuracy, there was a strong correlation between the predicted and actual survival, up to six months.
- Predictions of less than four weeks were the most precise (sometimes referred to as a "horizon effect").
- For predictions beyond six months, there was no relationship to actual survival. [29]

Some studies suggest an even greater distortion of reality: "Physicians' estimates of prognosis for patients in palliative care programs are overly optimistic by a factor of 3- to 5-fold—that is 300% to 500% more optimistic than observed. Other studies bolster the finding that physicians overestimate survival."[30]

Prognostic predictions are extremely important because "As the options for treating advanced cancer expand, it is crucial to identify not only those patients who will live long enough to benefit from therapy but also to avoid overly aggressive treatment in those who will not. Furthermore, patients base their treatment choices on their prognosis."[31] Yet, we've seen how these predictions can be quite flawed.

NOT CONFUSING STATISTICS FOR DETERMINANTS OF YOUR FUTURE

One should be careful not to confuse a personal prognosis with gross statistical averages for patients with certain types of cancer. Even so, some patients find value in examining the statistical survival data for their type of cancer. What follows is prognostic information for three commonly diagnosed cancers, which quickly demonstrates the level of variation in long-term outcome that occurs within cancer diagnoses. The following information is from the American Cancer Society:

- **Prognosis for Breast Cancer:** "Overall, 61% of breast cancer cases are diagnosed at a localized stage (no spread to lymph nodes or other locations outside the breast), for which the 5-year relative survival rate is 99%. If the cancer has spread to tissues or lymph nodes under the arm (regional stage), the survival rate is 84%. If the spread is to lymph nodes around the collarbone or to distant lymph nodes or organs (distant stage), the survival rate falls to 24%. For all stages combined, relative survival rates at 10 and 15 years after diagnosis are 83% and 78%, respectively."[32]
- **Prognosis for Lung Cancer:** "The 1- and 5-year relative survival rates for lung cancer cases diagnosed during 2003–2009 were 43% and 17%, respectively. Only 15% of lung cancers are diagnosed at a localized stage, for which the 5-year survival rate is 54%. The 5-year survival for small cell lung cancer (6%) is lower than that for non-small cell (18%)."[33]
- **Prognosis for Prostate Cancer:** "The majority (93%) of prostate cancers are discovered in the local or regional stages, for which the 5-year relative survival rate approaches 100%. Over the past 25 years, the 5-year relative survival rate for all stages combined has increased from 68% to almost 100%. According to the most recent data, 10- and 15-year relative survival rates are 99% and 94%, respectively."[34]

Whatever your prognosis is today, it can change over time and treatment. The world of cancer treatment is highly dynamic, and different doctors may prescribe different treatments, so it is important to have the right people on your team.

3

HOW TO SELECT YOUR DOCTORS AND TREATMENT FACILITIES

Myra C. has a great deal to say about physicians. Though not a doctor herself, Myra has devoted her life to advancing the field of bioethics. In 1982, she cofounded the Midwest Bioethics Center based on a profound interest in end-of-life issues and catalyzed by her mother's death from cancer. Forty years later, the Center for Practical Bioethics, as it is currently known, enjoys an international reputation for advocacy related to end-of-life and palliative care issues. Much of this is due to the indomitable spirit of Myra, which can be seen in the continuation of her story:

> The next morning [following surgery], when I spoke with the surgeon, we didn't do very well communicating with one another. I am not looking for a friend, but I am looking for a good doctor. He was abrupt. He said, "Because the tumor ruptured, you are going to need to start chemo as soon as possible."
>
> I said, "Well, maybe, but I'm not sure I will have chemo." He was very dismissive and said, "Don't be foolish. Of course you are going to have chemo!"
>
> It was really off-putting to me. I again said, "Maybe. Maybe not." I knew he and I were not going to do well with one another, so I told him I was going to shop around for an oncologist and figure out what to do.
>
> The next day while friends were visiting, in comes this kid. He taps on the door, and then just charges in, interrupting our conversa-

tion. He sits down, looking like he is all of twelve years old, and says, "I'm doctor so and so. I'm your oncologist."

I said, "I'm sorry. What did you just say?" He repeated himself, to which I replied, "Sweetheart, I'm sure you are an oncologist, but you are not *my* oncologist. So do you mind just leaving?"

Because of the work I do, I had lot of friends—great resources to turn to for information. I wanted to know everything in the world about my cancer. I read a lot. I knew I had a rare form of ovarian cancer that was very aggressive—its cells double at a rapid rate. I knew that I wanted to see someone who specialized in gynecological cancer, someone who was well trained, someone who was direct but not rude. So I began to ask people in Kansas City who would qualify. Dr. D.'s name surfaced several times.

I told a close friend who is an oncologist that I was thinking about Dr. D., and he said, "Wow, she's brilliant, top notch, and really strong willed and blunt and opinionated." My husband interrupted and said, "Bob, it sounds like Dr. D. and Myra would be fine together!" So I asked Bob if he would ask her to see me that week.

Dr. D. and I have done well together. We have our good days and bad days. Sometimes I tease her and ask her if she remembers the definition of shared decision making. I'm very fond of her.[1]

Myra offered this advice regarding the selection of your physician:

You want to know that your doctors are well trained. You want to talk to people who know your doctor. I also wanted someone who had published. I want to know not only the scientific data but what my doctor thinks about the problem—even though I may or may not pay attention to what she advises me to do.

I also think it is very important that it is someone that you can relate to. I wasn't looking for a good friend, but I did need to identify someone who would respect my role in treatment.

When you are talking about this journey, you're hopefully going to be with this person for a long time. That's why I believe in a covenantal approach to medicine—you can only be successful if each commits to the other.[2]

A TRUSTED GUIDE

Your doctors will serve as trusted guides throughout your cancer journey, so it is essential that you select physicians whom you trust and value. Few people know this better than Alta F., who has survived three separate cancer diagnoses during her seventy-four years of life. Her advice is simple: "You have to have faith in your doctor. If you have doubts, you are going to be in trouble."[3]

Most patients start the journey by consulting with their primary care physician (PCP). In many cases, he or she might be able to rule out cancer by appropriately attributing your symptoms to other, more benign causes. If cancer appears likely, your PCP will recommend a specialist, whose first job will be to render a definitive diagnosis and then suggest a treatment plan. That plan may include multiple other specialists—all of whom you will need to vet.

It may sound simple and straightforward, but here is where the path gets tricky. Before you accept your PCP's recommendations, you need to understand his or her thought process when referring you to a given specialist. There are numerous factors that can influence your doctor's recommendations, including:

- **The Role That Your PCP Wishes to Play in Your Treatment:** Some PCPs will quickly refer their patients to a specialist. Others may elect to order the initial imaging studies or other tests before determining whom you should see next.
- **The Type of Disease That Is Suspected:** Cancers of the blood would suggest an initial referral to a medical oncologist or hematologist, whereas a suspected solid tumor would likely result in an initial referral to a surgical specialist. More esoteric or rare tumors might justify a referral to a subspecialist known for his or her expertise in this particular disease.
- **The Various Cancer Specialists Who Are Available in Your Community:** The depth and breadth of cancer specialists varies dramatically across communities and health care institutions. If you live in a rural area or a small to midsized community, you may have to travel to receive disease-specific expertise. Your doctor will consider whether your functional status imposes any limita-

tions on travel. If not, he or she will help you weigh the potential trade-offs of leaving town for care.

- **The Hospital or Health System with Which Your PCP Is Aligned or Employed:** Physicians are often strongly encouraged to make referrals to colleagues within their own hospital or health care system. While financially beneficial to the health care organization, such practices are not necessarily in your best interest. Remember, not all doctors, including oncologists and surgeons, are equally competent.
- **Your Doctor's Historic Referral Patterns and Experiences, As Well As His or Her Biases:** We often give our PCP too much credit when it comes to discerning and utilizing the best referral sources available in the market. It is exceedingly difficult to differentiate among physicians based on clinical quality—unless the variation is blatant. Furthermore, they may simply lack exposure to specialists outside of their spheres of practice.

The key is finding the *right* doctor for you. For Lori and me, that meant someone with impeccable clinical skills, knowledge, and experience. We also wanted a doctor with whom we felt we had a trusted partnership—who was compassionate and a good communicator. Your list of virtues for the right physician may be different. The important thing is to have a list. Define what you are looking for in a specialist, and consider your first encounter with a new doctor like a job interview—with you conducting the interview.

UNDERSTANDING THE ROLE OF CANCER SPECIALISTS

Your chances of selecting the optimal specialists improve when you understand how to differentiate among doctors.

Lori and I believe it is helpful to first divide doctors into two major groups: (1) those specialists whose practices include—but do not treat exclusively—cancer patients, such as general surgeons, neurosurgeons, urologists, ENTs, and gynecologists, and (2) physicians whose sole focus is on cancer-related diagnoses. The second group, who are referred to as *oncologists*, can then be further divided into medical oncologists (who can also be trained as hematologists), radiation oncologists, and surgical oncologists.

Here's a short description of each specialty from the National Cancer Institute:

- **Medical Oncology** is a subspecialty of internal medicine. Doctors who specialize in internal medicine treat a wide range of medical problems. Medical oncologists treat cancer and manage the patient's course of treatment. A medical oncologist may also consult with other physicians about the patient's care or refer the patient to other specialists.
- **Hematology** is a subspecialty of internal medicine. Hematologists focus on diseases of the blood and related tissues, including the bone marrow, spleen, and lymph nodes.
- **Radiation Oncology** is a subspecialty of radiology. Radiology is the use of x-rays [*sic*] and other forms of radiation to diagnose and treat disease. Radiation oncologists specialize in the use of radiation to treat cancer.
- **Surgery** is a specialty that pertains to the treatment of disease by surgical operation. General surgeons perform operations on almost any area of the body. Surgeons can also choose to specialize in a certain type of surgery; for example, thoracic surgeons are specialists who perform operations specifically in the chest area, including the lungs and the esophagus. Oncologic surgeons specialize in operating on cancer.[4]

Medical, surgical, and radiation oncologists are required to pass comprehensive examinations in their specific fields, referred to as *boards*, in order to be *board certified*. Board certification is generally recognized as the minimum standard required to ensure that physicians possess the requisite level of clinical competency to practice in their specialties.

Medical, radiation, and surgical oncologists can be further differentiated based on their focuses on specific diseases or areas of the body. A surgical oncologist, for instance, can subspecialize in breast cancer. Though their knowledge about cancer is, by design, narrow, it can also be profoundly deep. One sees this division most commonly in large academic settings where oncologists possess even greater subspecialized training or experience.

Oncologists can complete formal training in their subspecialties, known as *fellowship training*. It is important to note that many physicians bestow upon themselves the title of *specialist* or *expert* in a given area, such as breast surgery, based on the volume of patients they treat for a specific condition. They can be experts, but before accepting their claims of expertise, it is perfectly acceptable to ask physicians about their formal training (i.e., are they fellowship trained?) and about their years of experience with patients who have conditions similar to yours.

WHAT DO YOU VALUE MOST IN A DOCTOR?

Now that you know how to differentiate among specialists based on their type of practice and level of training, it is time to consider other factors that can influence your selection process. Here is a quick list to get you started:

- **Participation in Your Insurance Plan.** Because of the extraordinary cost of health care services, the first screen that most people use when considering a physician is whether they participate in the patient's insurance plan. Unfortunately, some physicians may be inaccessible to you by virtue of being *out of network*—meaning that your insurance company has not contracted with these doctors to be part of their physician panel. Unless you are willing to pay heavily out of pocket, which can be financially devastating, you will need to find an in-network provider.
- **Reputation for Clinical Excellence.** Though it is difficult to quantify, every physician knows that there is tremendous variation in quality among doctors. There are ways to improve your probability of finding a clinically excellent doctor: (1) Begin by seeking out physicians who have a strong reputation within the community among both consumers and health care professionals—there is probably a good reason for them to be viewed positively. (2) Consider a physician who practices at a nationally recognized cancer center.
- **Training and Credentials.** Lori and I feel this issue bears repeating because the depth and breadth of a physician's training can also provide a proxy for quality. A basic starting point is to

ensure that your physician is board certified. You may then want to consider a physician who has received subspecialized training in the form of a fellowship. Some patients also consider where their physicians trained, believing that a fellowship from a prestigious cancer institute provides yet another level of assurance. As you go through this discernment process, please realize that there are also superlative physicians who do not possess these credentials.

- **Experience.** Nothing trumps the value of experience—and the insight, proficiency, and wisdom that can be gleaned through years of practice. Reams of data exist showing the correlation, for instance, between the number of surgical procedures performed by a physician and his or her outcomes. As Malcolm Gladwell discusses in his book *Outliers*, it generally takes a great deal of time to achieve mastery in any endeavor: "In fact, researchers have settled on what they believe is the magic number for true expertise: ten thousand hours."[5]

- **Alignment with a Specific Hospital or Health System.** Your physician is but one cog in the medical "machine" that provides care to cancer patients. The comprehensiveness, quality, and cutting-edge nature of this care will vary dramatically among free-standing centers, hospitals, and health systems. What may be available at your local community hospital could be a mere subset of the offerings at an academic medical center. Depending on your type of cancer, where you are treated could have a significant impact on your outcome. Remember, if your PCP is an employee of a hospital or health system, he or she is probably strongly encouraged to refer you to specialists within this system. That may or may not be in your best interest.

- **Referral Network.** It is important that, when selecting your first specialist, you have some sense of the other physicians to whom you may be referred. If your initial referral is to a surgeon, then he or she will likely have a preferred medical and radiation oncologist. Together, they will form your cancer treatment team. Ideally, you would want to conduct some level of due diligence on all of these doctors—but recognizing that timeliness of treatment can be important, that is probably not feasible. Therefore, there is even more reason for you to be comfortable with the system into which you are referred. It is essential that you are confident that all of the physicians meet a minimum standard of excellence.

- **Regular Participation in a Tumor Board.** Many cancer specialists attend regularly scheduled meetings in which a panel of diverse specialists review patients' findings and recommended treatment plans. It allows a specialist and their patients to receive a multidisciplinary review of their care and make any recommended course corrections. Lori and I feel strongly about the importance of tumor boards. We would consider making participation a prerequisite when selecting a specialist. Keep in mind, however, that the treatment of many early-stage cancers is so straightforward as to not warrant multidisciplinary review. Ask your specialist if he or she plans to present your case. If so, request a follow-up report on the consensus of the tumor board regarding your treatment.

- **Gender.** Whether you seek care from a male or female physician is primarily a matter of comfort for some patients. This issue most frequently comes into play in cases of breast cancer and genito-urinary tract diseases, such as cervical cancer.

- **Interpersonal Style.** The communication style and emotional intelligence of their physicians matters greatly to some patients and far less to others. Some patients simply want a physician with unquestionable clinical skills and are willing to defer to their physician's judgment. Others want to actively participate in treatment decisions and need a physician who is an extremely effective communicator, demonstrates clear empathy, and welcomes you as a partner on this journey. For patients facing a difficult prognosis, the emotional intelligence and emotional availability of their physicians can make a pronounced difference.

For readers interested in exploring these topics in more detail, consider reading my earlier book, *The Myths of Modern Medicine: The Alarming Truth about American Health Care*. Chapter 5 focuses exclusively on physician-related issues and elaborates on a number of the aforementioned topics.

IMPORTANT QUESTIONS TO ASK YOUR PCP ABOUT HIS REFERRAL RECOMMENDATION

The likelihood of finding a physician who meets your stringent qualifications increases dramatically when you become actively involved in the referral selection process. The specific action that you need to take is simple: Begin by asking your PCP a host of questions related to his recommendation, including:

- Why are you sending me to this type of specialist to make the diagnosis?
- What made you choose him or her over others in the field?
- If I wanted a second opinion from a physician at another hospital, to whom would you send me?

Your PCP should patiently answer your questions. If not, perhaps you need a new PCP. Let us assume that your physician is highly collaborative. Even so, do not feel pressured to accept his or her referral recommendation quite yet. It is perfectly acceptable to thank your doctor while indicating that you need a little more time to process the decision. Remember, despite the sense of urgency you are feeling, it is important to slow down long enough to make astute decisions. Only then are you empowered to take the right action.

OTHER SOURCES OF INFORMATION ABOUT PHYSICIANS

Now may be a good time to seek out other sources of information about appropriate specialists within your area. The trick when conducting such a search is to understand the relative validity of your sources before being swayed by the information they provide. Here are a few tips to get started:

- You may know doctors or nurses in the community. Health care workers can be a valuable source of information, but they bring obvious biases based on their experiences with specific providers and health systems. Nonetheless, I have learned a great deal from such sources, including surgical nurses who stand side by side with a plethora of surgeons in the OR. When they tell me that they would "not take their dog" to a given surgeon, you can bet I won't be taking my family member to him or her, either. Health care insiders can also articulate the positive points of differentiation for key specialists; for example, "He performs more than two hundred of these procedures each year and enjoys excellent clinical outcomes."

- The Internet offers robust information; unfortunately, much of it is of questionable validity. There are a host of trusted sites sponsored by major organizations, such as the National Cancer Institute, the Mayo Clinic, the American Cancer Society, National Cancer Care Network, and American College of Surgeons. Be cautious when reviewing sites focused on particular types of cancer—many of them are underwritten by pharmaceutical firms and are accordingly biased. We have included a list of resources at the end of the book that identifies trustworthy sources of information.

- When reviewing content on hospital or health system sites, take all stated claims with a grain of salt. Much of it is marketing hyperbole and can bear little resemblance to the truth. Also be wary of sites that purportedly rate the quality of physicians. Such sites are in their infancy and hence are of questionable value. Their ratings are often predicated upon patient evaluations of the nonclinical attributes of care, for example, whether the physician was nice. You may, however, be able to access important biographical information about a physician, including education, training, certifications, and years in practice via the Internet.

The National Cancer Institute offers the following recommendations for finding the right physician for you:

- Your local hospital or its patient referral service may be able to provide you with a list of specialists who practice at that hospital.
- The American Board of Medical Specialties (ABMS) has a list of doctors who have met certain education and training requirements and have passed specialty examinations.
- The American Medical Association (AMA) DoctorFinder database provides basic information on licensed physicians in the United States. Users can search for physicians by name or by medical specialty.

- The American Society of Clinical Oncology (ASCO) provides an online list of doctors who are members of ASCO. The member database has the names and affiliations of nearly 30,000 oncologists worldwide. It can be searched by doctor's name, institution, location, oncology specialty, and/or type of board certification.
- The American College of Surgeons (ACS) membership database is an online list of surgeons who are members of the ACS. The list can be searched by doctor's name, geographic location, or medical specialty. The ACS can be contacted by telephone at 1-800-621-4111.
- The American Osteopathic Association (AOA) Find a Doctor database provides an online list of practicing osteopathic physicians who are AOA members. The information can be searched by doctor's name, geographic location, or medical specialty. The AOA can be contacted by telephone at 1-800-621-1773.
- Local medical societies may maintain lists of doctors in each specialty.
- Public and medical libraries may have print directories of doctors' names listed geographically by specialty.
- Your nearest NCI-designated cancer center can provide information about doctors who practice at that center. The NCI-Designated Cancer Centers' Find a Cancer Center page provides contact information to help health care providers and cancer patients with referrals to NCI-designated cancer centers located throughout the United States.[6]

Lori also suggests that the American Society for Therapeutic Radiation Oncology can be a valuable resource for information related to radiation oncology and its practitioners.

IDENTIFYING THE RIGHT FACILITIES TO DIAGNOSE AND TREAT YOUR DISEASE

When you select a physician, you are de facto selecting the facilities at which he or she practices. Because not all cancer facilities are comparable, it is important to understand your physician's affiliations. In fact, facilities that treat cancer vary dramatically in their capabilities, treatment volumes, clinical outcomes, and patient satisfaction.

Among the most comprehensive cancer centers are those bearing an NCI designation:

> The NCI-designated cancer centers program recognizes centers around the country that meet rigorous criteria for world-class, state-of-the-art programs in multidisciplinary cancer research. These centers put significant resources into developing research programs, faculty, and facilities that will lead to better approaches to prevention, diagnosis, and treatment of cancer. The NCI designation not only recognizes excellence but opens doors to greater federal funding, information sharing, and resources.[7]

There are sixty-eight NCI-designated facilities, the vast majority of which are academic medical centers.

There is a further division within NCI-designated centers, noted by adding the word *comprehensive* to the name. Only about 60 percent of the NCI-designated cancer centers are comprehensive cancer centers. For a center to earn this distinction, it must

> demonstrate reasonable depth and breadth of research in each of three major areas: laboratory, clinical, and population-based research, as well as substantial transdisciplinary research that bridges these scientific areas. In addition, a comprehensive center must also demonstrate professional and public education and outreach capabilities, including the dissemination of clinical and public health advances in the communities it serves.[8]

Though these facilities generally have tremendous capabilities, NCI-designated centers are not right for everyone, as was the case with Myra:

> A lot of people have asked me why I did not go to a National Cancer Institute-designated center and instead saw a physician in a private hospital. My mom died of cancer and received care in an academic institution. She received excellent care, but that whole model of care in which students are coming in and out is a different model. The focus is on research and training, with patient care being third. Frankly, I wanted people focused on me—not their next publication.[9]

There are many exemplary cancer treatment facilities without NCI designation. The NCI suggests a series of questions to help determine if a treatment facility is right for you:

- Has the facility had experience and success in treating my condition?
- Has the facility been rated by state, consumer, or other groups for its quality of care?
- How does the facility check on and work to improve its quality of care?
- Has the facility been approved by a nationally recognized accrediting body, such as the ACS Commission on Cancer and/or The Joint Commission?
- Does the facility explain patients' rights and responsibilities? Are copies of this information available to patients?
- Does the treatment facility offer support services, such as social workers and resources, to help me find financial assistance if I need it?
- Is the facility conveniently located?[10]

In addition to NCI designation, two other resources can aid you in your search for the right facility. The American Cancer Society's Commission on Cancer has identified more than 1,430 treatment facilities in the United States that offer approved programs. These programs have been vetted to ensure that they fulfill the criteria associated with delivering quality cancer care. A complete list of these programs can be found on the ACS website. You can also contact the Commission on Cancer by telephone at (312) 202-5085 or by e-mail at CoC@facs.org.

Finally, you may wish to contact the Joint Commission:

> The Joint Commission is an independent not-for-profit organization that evaluates and accredits health care organizations and programs in the United States. It also offers information for the general public about choosing a treatment facility. The Joint Commission can be contacted by telephone at 630-792-5000. The Joint Commission offers an online Quality Check service that patients can use to determine whether a specific facility has been accredited by the Joint Commission and to view the organization's performance reports.[11]

Remember, if you are a member of a health insurance plan, your choice of treatment facilities may be limited to those that participate in your plan. Your insurance company can provide you with a list of approved facilities. Nurses and social workers may also be able to provide you with more information about coverage, eligibility, and insurance issues. Although the costs of cancer treatment can be very high, you do have the option of paying out of pocket if you want to use a treatment facility that is not covered by your insurance plan. If you are considering paying for treatment yourself, you may wish to discuss the possible costs with a financial counselor associated with your doctor's office prior to treatment.

DETERMINING WHETHER LOCAL RESOURCES ARE ADEQUATE TO MEET YOUR NEEDS

Most cancer patients will find all of the needed resources for their journeys within their own communities. However, some patients may need to seek care at facilities geographically distant from home. Some of the primary reasons for considering traveling for care include:

- the diagnosis of a condition that is either relatively rare or for which there is no well-defined standard of care,
- the presence of complicating medical conditions that impact your ability to receive the standard of care,
- concerns over the quality of care available in your community,
- the desire to see a recognized expert in the particular condition from which you suffer,
- a desire for some level of anonymity while going through treatment, and
- the availability of selective clinical trials (that may not be available in your community).

Some patients elect to leave home to obtain a second opinion, a topic we explore in more detail in chapter 7. Many of these patients then have the prescribed therapies administered by local clinicians.

Before you elect to leave home for care, it is important that you recognize some of the difficulties you will likely encounter. You can weigh the pros and cons before deciding what is in your best interest:

- There may be significant financial implications of your decision based on insurance and costs associated with travel and lodging for your family.
- By being away from home, your support network could be diminished.
- You may miss the comfort and familiarity of home while undergoing difficult treatments at a facility that is foreign to you.
- You could have more trouble navigating between various providers in an unfamiliar city.
- Continuity of care may be more difficult once you return home.

OVERCOMING FINANCIAL BARRIERS TO TRAVEL

Some patients may have difficulty bearing the burden of travel expense associated with seeking care outside of their communities. Fortunately, there are organizations that provide assistance with travel costs, including but not limited to:

- Air Charity Network,
- Corporate Angel Network,
- Joe's House,
- Ronald McDonald House Charities, and
- Hope Lodge (American Cancer Society).

DECIDING ON A DOCTOR AND FACILITY

Regardless of the scope of your search, once you feel that you've conducted an adequate due diligence, it's time to make a decision, share your conclusions with your PCP, and ask him or her for help in expediting the scheduling of your first appointment.

When you meet with the selected specialist, again view it as a job interview in which you are interviewing the doctor. You've evaluated him or her in absentia, but now that you are actively interacting, are you happy with your choice? If so, listen carefully to his or her recommendations on the plan to treat your cancer. If not, take the time to start over; chances are there were one or two "runners-up" in your selection process.

CAVEAT EMPTOR

It is important that you and your family be able to differentiate between unsubstantiated marketing claims by certain cancer facilities and the truth. Lori and I cringe when we see warm television ads promising comprehensive care, unique treatment modalities, and great outcomes regardless of the nature of one's diagnosis.

Every cancer patient wants the best chance at recovery and deserves to receive it. Some cancer facilities, however, may be more adept at tailoring their marketing messages than delivering clinically superior care. Truly exemplary facilities may do a modicum of advertising, but they do not make exaggerated claims. Rather, they build their reputation daily, patient by patient, predicated on the excellence of their care. Be careful not to be misled by false claims at a time when you or a loved one is extremely vulnerable and searching for the best care.

A FINAL NOTE OF CAUTION

Myra offers an important cautionary note to patients entering the health care system:

> One piece of advice I would offer is that you have to take control of your situation. Our health care system is in disarray. Right now it is a mess. Either you or someone close to you has to advocate for you. Health care is a pretty hostile territory. People wander in having no idea what can happen to them. This sounds so awful, but I sometimes think about the lamb to slaughter. Granted, there are miracles that happen every day in our health care system, and there are wonderful people who work within it. But the system is stacked against the patient. The patient has to figure out how to manage it. They cannot rely on their physician for this task. [12]

These words likely sound unduly harsh—particularly at a time when you need to put great trust in the providers from whom you will receive care. They are not harsh; they are the reality of today's health care system.

4

GENETIC TESTING IN DIAGNOSIS AND TREATMENT

Even as a small child, Mary E. knew she wanted to be a nurse someday. After completing nursing school, Mary spent the first half of her career working on both rehab and medical-surgical units of a hospital. It was oncology nursing, though, that would capture Mary's heart and give her life a tremendous sense of purpose.

Day in and day out, as Mary cared for her cancer patients, she had no awareness that locked deep within her genes was a secret—a small change in the genetic code that would predispose her to cancer.

Her cancer journey began at a tumultuous time in her life:

> I was divorced in September and then went for my routine mammogram in October. That was on a Friday, after which I took off for Minnesota to celebrate my divorce with my best friend, who had been my maid of honor during my wedding. She had also lent me money during my divorce. While up there, I got a call saying that I needed to come back for an ultrasound. After working in oncology for so many years, I knew exactly what that meant.
>
> As soon as I got back, I went in for the ultrasound. They then said I needed a biopsy. Meanwhile, I was communicating with the people I knew in radiation oncology at St. Mary's, who kept reassuring me that I was fine. But I had a premonition—a dream. Whenever something big happens in my life, my dad comes to me. In the dream, it was not quite winter, but it was cold out. He had a very serious look

on his face. I didn't want to hear what he had to say, so I woke myself up. I knew he was going to warn me.

They did a biopsy. Someone had told me that that if you watch the biopsy on the screen, when the needle penetrates the mass, it will collapse if it is a cyst. If it doesn't, it's probably cancer. I watched, and it didn't collapse. I said, "Oh shit!"

My primary care called to tell me, but I had already looked up the results. It was a very small tumor, maybe 5 millimeters. I was stage 1.[1]

Thanks to early detection, Mary's cancer was easily treated with breast-conserving surgery (lumpectomy) followed by radiation and hormonal therapy. Her medical oncologist, Dr. E., recommended genetic testing on the small chance that Mary would carry the BRCA genetic mutation. Unfortunately, because of the low incidence of BRCA mutations in patients under fifty, Mary's insurance company would not cover the cost at the time.

As someone newly divorced, Mary was living paycheck to paycheck—which made the $2,000 out-of-pocket expense for testing out of the question. Mary took comfort in the fact that she did not fit the typical demographic profile for BRCA, which disproportionately affects women of Jewish ancestry from eastern Europe. Still, a niggling seed of doubt had been planted in her mind—a seed that was about to germinate.

About a year later, I was attending a presentation on genetics by Dr. G. He said that any woman under the age of fifty diagnosed with breast cancer should be tested for a genetic mutation. He said that insurance companies were now paying for the test. So at my next appointment with Dr. E., I said, "I have a different insurance plan now. Can we try again?" We did, and it was covered.

I found out that I carried the BRCA2 gene, which is the rarer of the two BRCA genes. It increases the risk of ovarian cancer, colon cancer, breast cancer, and melanoma. When we discussed it and found out that I was positive, we thought there must be some Jewish ancestry, which is surprising and not. My family is from eastern Europe. My father was from far-western Ukraine. In fact, he lived in an area that was so far west that, depending upon who won the last war, he was either Ukrainian or Polish. My mother was from a different part of Ukraine.[2]

Mary's father served in Hitler's army in World War II. Unlike Mary, he had little tolerance for people of different faiths—particularly Jews. Therefore, Mary, who is wonderfully devoid of any such prejudices, joked, "The thing I'm going say to my father [in the afterlife], who was so anti-Semitic, so prejudiced, is, 'Listen, buddy, there was some Jewish person mucking around with some non-Jewish person in our family because I've got the proof!'"

THE EMERGING GENETIC REVOLUTION IN MEDICINE

There has been phenomenal growth in our understanding of the underlying causes of many types of cancer. While some cancers are linked to environmental factors, ranging from exposure to certain viruses to mutagenic chemicals, other cancers are proving to be genetically linked. In fact, "more than 200 hereditary cancer susceptibility syndromes have been described. . . . Although many of these are rare syndromes, they are thought to account for at least 5–10% of all cancer."[3] These genetic mutations may be linked to breast, ovarian, colon, and a broad number of other types of cancer.

Genetic mutations appear to exert varying levels of influence on the development of certain types of cancer. The strength of this influence varies considerably based on the genetic anomaly. These genetic defects could result in cancers that appear in seemingly unrelated parts of the body. The same genetic defect underlying some breast cancers, for instance, could also trigger the development of ovarian cancer.

An understanding of one's genetic profile, and hence known risks for developing cancer, allows physicians to recommend not only preventative measures but also a new, expanding armamentarium of treatments that seek to control the cancer through an understanding of the specific genetic defect.

GENETIC COUNSELING AND RISK ASSESSMENT

After completing your medical history and physical examination, your physician may recommend genetic counseling. "Genetic counseling and risk assessment is the process of identifying and counseling individuals at increased risk of developing cancer, and distinguishing between those at high risk . . . those at modestly increased risk . . . and those at average risk."[4]

The most basic form of genetic screening examines the history of cancer within your family, usually going back three to four generations. This information allows for the creation of a family chart that identifies all known instances of cancer in immediate relatives. A genetic counselor then looks for patterns of cancer occurrence. These patterns may be of seemingly unrelated diseases, such as ovarian cancer and breast cancer, yet they could share a common genetic defect. As our knowledge of the genetic basis of cancer increases, so, too, will our ability to screen effectively.

The genetic counselor may also factor other, more specific information into your risk profile:

> There are a number of family history factors that can be indicative of increased cancer risk and can guide risk assessment. These include multiple close relatives with similar or related cancer, early age at diagnosis, an individual having more than one primary tumor or bilateral cancers in paired organs, the presence of rare cancer or tumors, ethnicity, and individuals with unusual or excessive benign lesions (such as colon polyps, dysplastic moles, or rare adrenal tumors.[5]

Your physician may also utilize web-based tools to aid assessing your risk, including the U.S. Surgeon General's Family Health Portrait tool (http://www.hhs.gov/familyhistory).

The American Cancer Society also provides a simple checklist to help determine if you may benefit from genetic testing. Such testing may be indicated if any of the following statements are true for you:

- Several first-degree relatives (mother, father, sisters, brothers, children) with cancer, especially the same type of cancer
- Cancers in your family that are sometimes linked to a single gene mutation (for instance, breast, ovarian, and pancreatic cancer)
- Family members who had cancer at a younger age than normal for that type of cancer
- Close relatives with rare cancers that are linked to inherited cancer syndromes

- A physical finding that is linked to an inherited cancer (such as having many colon polyps)
- A known genetic mutation in one or more family members who have already had genetic testing[6]

For some people, like Mary, it is almost impossible to reconstruct their family history: "I don't know anything about my ancestors beyond my parents. My dad's father may have died of cancer, but they lived in a small Ukrainian village, so who knows what the diagnosis was?"[7] For such patients, genetic testing becomes the next step.

GENETIC TESTING

When screening suggests that a patient could be at risk for a genetic abnormality, his or her blood or saliva sample can be sent to a specialized laboratory for analysis. The blood is tested for a panel of genetic abnormalities that represent known risk factors for cancer. One of the best known of such abnormalities is a defect in the BRCA1 and BRCA2 genes.

Other forms of genetic tests are also emerging. On August 11, 2014, the FDA approved a genetic test through the screening of stool samples designed to identify abnormalities that may contribute to the development of colon cancer.[8] The test, marketed as Cologuard by its developer, Exact Sciences, has yet to be proven effective in the field. If, however, it lives up to expectations, it may become a potent, noninvasive way of identifying people at risk for colon cancer.

THE RISKS ASSOCIATED WITH BEING BRCA-POSITIVE

There are two known mutations of the BRCA gene, referred to as BRCA1 and BRCA2. As previously mentioned, these mutations are most commonly found in a subpopulation referred to as Ashkenazi Jews—Jewish people with familial roots in central and eastern Europe—though others can be affected. Women with this mutation are at far greater risk for developing breast and ovarian cancer.

Though estimates range widely, most experts agree that the increased risk of developing breast and ovarian cancer is substantial:

A woman with a deleterious gene mutation predisposing her to cancer, such as in BRCA1 or BRCA2, and who does not have a personal diagnosis of cancer, has a 60–85% risk of breast cancer in her lifetime compared to a woman of average breast cancer risk who has approximately a 12% lifetime risk. Additionally, while 1.4% of American women will have an ovarian cancer diagnosis in their lifetime, 15–40% of women with a deleterious BRCA1 or BRCA2 gene mutation will receive an ovarian cancer diagnosis.[9]

In addition to far greater incidence rates, "Women with these mutations are four to five times more likely to develop aggressive breast cancers, according to the National Cancer Institute. The disease often comes at an early age and in both breasts."[10]

Because of the high statistical probability of developing cancer, many BRCA-positive women opt for preventative treatment, including prophylactic bilateral (double) mastectomies, as well as removal of their ovaries. These are difficult decisions for many reasons, including potential changes to one's body image, sexuality, and the onset of menopause.

Had Mary known about her BRCA status at the time of diagnosis, she may well have opted for a mastectomy versus a lumpectomy. Now, facing the specter of a potential cancer recurrence, Mary has yearly MRI scans of her breasts. She also had her ovaries prophylactically removed to prevent a threat of another cancer.

BRCA IS NOT THE ONLY GENETIC ABERRATION CONFERRING RISK

We are on the very cusp of discovering the role that numerous genetic mutations play in increasing the probability of certain types of cancer. While a spotlight has been shone on BRCA due to its clear correlation with breast and other types of cancer, new studies are revealing the potent role of other genes in cancer formation, including PALB2.

In a study published in the August 7, 2014, issue of the prestigious *New England Journal of Medicine*, the incidence of cancer was examined among 362 individuals with mutations of the PALB2 gene.[11] The study concluded that, depending on an individual's age, the increased probability of developing breast cancer due to this genetic mutation was up to nine times that of the normal female population. The largest increase in relative risk was found in women under the age of forty.[12] Just as BRCA was not the end of the story, neither is PALB2.

Genetic mutations play a role in the formation of numerous types of cancer beyond breast cancer. One example can be seen in patients afflicted with Lynch syndrome, an inherited disorder that may contribute to the potential development of specific types of cancer. Of the 140,000 new cases of colon cancer diagnosed each year, approximately 3 to 5 percent are attributable to Lynch-related genetic mutations. Beyond colon and rectal cancers, Lynch syndrome is also associated with an increased risk of numerous other types of cancer, ranging from ovarian to brain cancer.[13] A positive diagnosis of Lynch syndrome allows patients to be closely monitored via an array of screening modalities. In some cases, surgeries, such as hysterectomies, can be performed prophylactically.[14]

The National Institutes of Health publishes detailed information about various cancers for which there are known genetic links. This information is organized by type of cancer and can be found at http://www.cancer.gov/cancertopics/genetics.

THE IMPORTANCE OF INFORMED CONSENT

The National Society of Genetic Counselors advises that, prior to undergoing genetic testing, it is essential that you understand a number of variables, including:

- what specific tests are being proposed and why;
- the "benefits, risks, and limitations" of the tests;
- how the results can impact not only the patient but also his or her family members;
- how the information might be misused despite efforts to legislatively limit the potential for genetic discrimination; and
- alternatives to genetic testing.[15]

Prior to undergoing any type of preventative surgery, informed consent would mandate that the patient understand:

- the anticipated benefit of the surgery;
- potential side effects and risks associated with the surgery;

- ancillary concerns, such as the financial impact of treatment; and
- an accurate assessment of the risks associated with forgoing surgery.

ETHICAL ISSUES ASSOCIATED WITH SCREENING AND TESTING

The genetic profiling of patients raises numerous ethical issues, starting with the ramifications of sharing genetic risk information within the family. If, for instance, a patient tests positive for a genetic abnormality, such as BRCA, is there an obligation to inform the patient's children (who might be adults) that they are also at risk? Imagine that you are the twenty-one-year-old daughter of a BRCA-positive mother who is learning for the first time that she, too, may carry a defective gene that will almost surely mandate facing some very difficult life decisions related to preventative surgeries.

Mary initially struggled when it came to telling her children:

> I told my kids . . . starting with my daughter. I started crying—not because I was scared—I wasn't scared—but because I didn't want to cause her pain.
>
> I told my children that they each had a 50-50 risk of carrying the gene. It is now up to them to decide what they want to do. My daughter has told me that she does not want to know her status. She is going to start her mammograms at the age of thirty-seven.
>
> I told her, even if you find out that you carry the gene, don't let it affect your life. I had two beautiful children who I'm so grateful I brought into this world. Everyone has something![16]

In recent years, some high profile BRCA-positive patients, such as actress Angelina Jolie, have spoken up about their genetic status, as well as their preventative surgeries. There are two positive aspects to this phenomenon: (1) It helps destigmatize such procedures as bilateral mastectomies, and (2) it increases awareness that women may be at risk for a BRCA-related cancer. The ethical conundrum lies in an unintended consequence whereby women who are neither BRCA-positive nor have an aggressive breast tumor opt for radical surgeries when far more minor procedures would have the same outcome.

As our knowledge of the genetic basis of diseases increases and the cost of performing genetic analyses falls, there is a growing fear of genetic discrimination on the part of employers or insurers:

> About 700,000 Americans have had their DNA sequenced, in full or in part, and the number is rising rapidly as costs plummet—to $1,000 or less for a full genome, down from more than $1 million less than a decade ago.
>
> But many people are avoiding the tests because of a major omission in the 2008 federal law that bars employers and health insurers from seeking the results of genetic testing.
>
> The Genetic Information Nondiscrimination Act, known as GINA, does not apply to three types of insurance—life, disability, and long-term care—that are especially important to people who may have serious inherited diseases. Sponsors of the act say that they were well aware of the omission, but after a 14-year effort to write and pass the law, they had to settle for what they could get.
>
> That leaves many patients who may be at risk for inherited diseases fearful that a positive result could be used against them.[17]

Another ethical conundrum is who should bear the cost of preventative treatments for genetic defects. Not only is this an issue in the United States, where health care costs are the highest per capita in the world, but also in such countries as Israel, where as many as 1 million women may be at risk.[18]

DELAY OF TREATMENT CAUSED BY GENETIC TESTING

Genetic testing requires patience. It is not yet rapid. The results typically take weeks to receive. Patients and their physicians who are anxious to initiate treatment can find waiting for genetic results to be problematic. However, the results could change the course of treatment. Take the stage 1 breast cancer patient, for example. Without evidence of an underlying genetic abnormality, she can safely elect for breast-conserving surgery (lumpectomy). However, if she proves to be BRCA-positive, her surgeon is probably going to recommend mastectomies. Does she wait for the results or proceed with the minimally invasive lumpectomy knowing that there may be a need to return for surgery that is more aggressive? These issues compound the high level of anxiety already being experienced by the newly diagnosed cancer patient.

THE GENETIC PROFILE OF YOUR TUMOR

Just as scientists can examine your DNA, they can also examine the DNA of your tumor. Such analysis provides important clues as to the relative aggressiveness of the tumor, as well as potential pathways for blocking the growth or even survival of the tumor. An example of such tumor genetic profiling can be seen in Oncotype DX:

> A 21-gene test called Oncotype DX can be performed on the tumor tissue to help with decision making about chemotherapy. The 21-gene test evaluates the genetic makeup of the tumor and provides a number score to help predict the chance of recurrence. The score is called the "recurrence score" and the results range from 1 to 100. Women with estrogen receptor positive, node negative breast cancer that have low recurrence scores will not need chemotherapy while women with high scores may benefit from chemotherapy. This test is only appropriate for women with estrogen receptor positive tumors.[19]

Lori's oncologist recommended an Oncotype DX analysis of her tumor and told us that a recurrence score above 23 would indicate the probable need for chemotherapy. We were extraordinarily relieved when the recurrence score proved to be less than 10.

GENETIC COUNSELING AS AN ONGOING COMPONENT OF TREATMENT

Though the current health care system is set up to deliver genetic services over a limited period of time, research reveals that "Instead of providing all of the complex medical information required of a typical genetic counseling session in one sitting, participants in this study sought more long term comprehensive care that evolved as their specific needs and experiences evolved."[20]

AS OUR UNDERSTANDING OF CANCER CHANGES, SO, TOO, DO OUR TREATMENTS

Our increasing knowledge of the role of genetics in cancer will ultimately usher in a revolution in personalized medicine. Signs of the revolution are abundant, and scientific breakthroughs are happening at a dizzying pace. However, it will still be decades before our reliance on the standard modalities of surgery, chemotherapy, and radiation for many cancer patients changes.

SOME PARTING WORDS OF ADVICE FROM OUR BRCA-POSITIVE PATIENT

Mary, who offers the unique perspective of being an oncology nurse who is BRCA-positive, gives some simple yet profound advice: "Some people allow the illness to envelope them; it defines them and their lives. I want to say, 'You have a whole life, and this is not your life.' Every day we get closer to our death. It is what you do with the time you have left. Be proactive. Take charge of your life. Don't hide from what is there!"[21]

5

MAKING SENSE OF YOUR TREATMENT OPTIONS

Stephen M. had done his homework. As a college professor, he was comfortable vigorously researching topics of interest—including a newly identified threat to his life. After much reading and investigation, he understood the risks, treatment options, and potential outcomes associated with his relatively early-stage prostate cancer:

> My urologist indicated that the biopsy results suggested that I was not a good candidate for active surveillance. He explained some of the options but pushed the prostatectomy because that's what urologists do. One thing that I worry about is the fact that you seem to get the advice from various specialists to pursue the type of care their specialty delivers.
>
> My inclination was to think more of active surveillance as a legitimate mode of treatment. I was thinking of it as a treatment versus not doing anything. In my mind, there was a question as to whether this is a disease that has to be treated or more a comment on natural aging. I certainly have been aware of the issues associated with screening and overtreatment.
>
> My GP was helpful in sorting through treatment options. One advantage that I had was that prostate cancer is not rapid growing, unlike cancers where you have to act very quickly. I had time and took the time.
>
> My base position was active surveillance. If I was advising people, I would tell them that's where you need to start. The question then becomes, When do you decide to treat?

In addition to talking with friends who are doctors, I sought out some friends and colleagues who had prostate cancer treatment.

From what I had read, I really wanted to avoid a prostatectomy due to side effects. In my mind, the first question was efficacy. Then the second question was side effects. And, to some extent, the third question would focus on convenience and those sorts of things.

For my cancer, there appeared to be no difference in treatment outcome between the major types of treatment, so I started going down the list of additional questions. With brachytherapy [implanted radioactive seeds], it was one outpatient procedure versus eight weeks of radiation therapy.

I'm very grateful that the three doctors I worked most closely with did not push any particular type of therapy. Everyone was willing to let me make my own decision.

I thought that brachytherapy had some very attractive options, but there was some question as to whether or not I qualified for it. My staging was a T2, but it was almost a T3. Dr. S. assured me that I did qualify for it. I then went to Lori (Dr. Lori Lindstrom Leifer) to ask her opinion regarding the brachytherapy. She also assured me that it was an appropriate way to go.

Both Lori and Dr. S. agreed that an MRI would be a smart move, so I went ahead and did that. The MRI showed that my disease was confined to the prostate, but there was enough in there to consider treating. The carcinoma was butting up against the wall of the prostate. It was the MRI that made it pretty clear that now was the time for treatment. I didn't want to risk it spreading outside of the prostate.

I felt quite comfortable with my decision. I had gone back to the people I trusted, which made me feel confident I was doing the right thing. I also did my own research, looking at a variety of different sources. You can do overkill—there is a point at which you know enough to make a good decision.[1]

A REMINDER TO SLOW DOWN: TAKING TIME TO UNDERSTAND YOUR TREATMENT OPTIONS

Every cancer patient reaches a point early in the journey when they must make decisions regarding treatment. For some cancer patients, there is one well-established protocol for the treatment of the disease.

However, for the majority of cancers, there are often different paths that physicians and patients can pursue in seeking to halt the spread of the disease.

Stephen waited ten months between initial diagnosis and commencing treatment. No layperson could have been better prepared intellectually to weigh the pros and cons of various treatment options than Stephen. Yet, that did not make the decision any easier. He did the smart thing: He took his foot off the accelerator and granted himself time to slow down.

That's exactly what the American Cancer Society advises: "Most cancers do not grow very quickly, so there's usually plenty of time to get information about the cancer, see specialists, and make decisions about what treatment option is best."[2] Karen Sepucha, the Harvard-based researcher we met earlier, echoes this sentiment: "Although cancer is serious, it is not usually an emergency. If people are in a panic mode, a lot of the skills that they bring to bear, or assets that allow them to make decisions, get thrown out the window. So I think we need to help patients get out of the panic mode so that they can absorb information and really participate in decisions. My advice is to take some time."[3]

Sepucha goes on to point out, "Medicine is not an exact science. There is rarely one right answer that works for every patient, so patients need to make sure that they are not waiting for their doctor to tell them what to do, thinking that there is some form of test that is going to tell them exactly what is right for them."[4]

BEING AWARE OF THE POTENTIAL BIASES OF SPECIALISTS

Stephen M. discovered that some physicians can reflect the biases of their specialties when making treatment recommendations. Though not surprising, it is a profoundly important thought because by pursuing one course of action, patients often negate other options.

Sepucha puts it this way:

> They need to be aware that, if they are going to see a surgeon, they are likely to hear about surgery. If they are going to a radiation oncologist, they are likely to hear about radiation. And that they need

to be the one to ensure that they hear all of the different views because it is not often the case that the doctor will share everything.

We've worked with a lot of doctors, and they will say, "Well, they know I'm a radiation oncologist—that's why they are coming to me, to hear about what I do. So why would I talk to them about some other things? This is what I know, this is what I do, and they are in my office." So they are making the assumption that the patient is in their office to talk about their specialty.[5]

Earlier, we mentioned the importance of having physicians who regularly participate in multidisciplinary tumor boards. One of the reasons for this strong recommendation is that the presentation of patients' cases in such conferences can help correct for the treatment biases that naturally exist within specialties.

PATIENT, KNOW THYSELF

Before mentally sorting through treatment options, Sepucha advises that patients need to understand and communicate what is important to them in the context of their lives:

We are asking patients to do their homework, which is different than showing up at the doctor's office and expecting the doctor to tell you what to do. The homework is not just on the medical stuff but on who you are, what you are about, and how you convey that in a way that is acceptable to the physician. Patients are the only ones who can communicate this type of information.[6]

Once their homework is completed, patients are ready to engage in a discussion with their physicians about the goals of treatment.

ESTABLISHING THE GOALS OF TREATMENT

Once there is an agreement on diagnosis and prognosis, you and your physician will explore treatment options based upon the goals of treatment:

Depending on your cancer type and stage, your goals for treatment might be:

- **Cure.** When you're first diagnosed, it's likely you'll be interested in treatments that cure cancer. When a cure is possible, you may be willing to endure more short-term side effects in return for the chance at a cure.
- **Control.** If your cancer is at a later stage or if previous treatments have been unsuccessful, you might adjust your goal to controlling your cancer. Different treatments may attempt to temporarily shrink or stop your cancer from growing. If this is your goal, you might not be willing to endure the side effects of harsher treatments.
- **Comfort.** If you have an advanced stage of cancer or one that hasn't responded to treatments, you might decide that comfort is most important to you. You and your doctor will work together to make sure you are free of pain and other symptoms.[7]

An essential division within prognoses is between cancers that are curable and those that are responsive to treatment but not curable. The term *incurable* once suggested a hasty and often unpleasant death, but thanks to advancements in medical science and the resulting plethora of new treatment modalities, many "incurable" cancers behave more like chronic conditions.

Patients may live with such conditions for decades, even though the disease can never be fully eradicated from their bodies. Such was the case with Patricia H., as recounted by her husband, Darrell: "We had an experience with a veteran oncology nurse at Saint Luke's. One day, while she was watching over Patricia, she said, 'You know lymphoma is the darnedest thing. It's very easy to slow it down, but it's almost impossible to cure it.' That was, in some ways, a great relief; it sounds more like a chronic disease than a life-threatening disease—just have to keep knocking it down."[8]

One of the terms you may hear frequently is *remission*. Patients, family, and friends may equate the term with "cure," which may or may not be accurate:

> Remission is a period of time when the cancer is responding to treatment or is under control. In a complete remission, all the signs and symptoms of the disease go away and cancer cells cannot be

found with any of the tests available for that cancer. It's also possible to have a partial remission. This is when the cancer shrinks but does not completely disappear. Remissions can last anywhere from many weeks to many years. Complete remissions may go on for years and over time be considered cures. If the cancer returns, more treatment can lead to another remission. A cancer that has recurred (come back) may respond to a different type of treatment, such as a different drug combination or radiation versus surgery.[9]

Three-time cancer survivor Alta F. describes a chronic state of cancer quite succinctly: "People will say to me, 'Oh, you're cured,' and I say, 'No. You are never cured. I'm in remission.'"

DETERMINING THE APPROPRIATENESS OF TREATMENT

Whether your treatment is intended to cure you, extend your life, or offer comfort, it is important to avoid misunderstandings that could adversely impact your ability to make informed decisions regarding your care. Such decisions can result in unnecessary or futile care that adversely impacts your quality of life but not your prognosis. Beyond the human toll, there is also an unnecessary financial burden imposed by inappropriate care. Yet, despite the importance for patients to be fully informed, the research clearly shows how many patients remain in the dark when it comes to their disease:

Among a group of 181 patients diagnosed with advanced cancer and receiving palliative care, for example, Craft, Burns, Smith, and Broom (2005) found that only 45% correctly understood their terminal status and the goals for treatment. Similarly, Chan and Woodruff (1997) report that among 131 patients with advanced malignancy, approximately 10% did not know they had cancer and 33% were unclear about the long-term prognosis.[10]

We found that approximately 25% of patients did not appear to understand the goals of the potentially toxic chemotherapy they were receiving. Patient and physician clarity at the time of treatment decision-making regarding GOC [goals of care] is of critical importance given that misunderstandings such as these have the potential to lead to future requests for more intense, but often futile chemotherapy.[11]

Sepucha notes,

> Often the hope gets tied to the next treatment and whether it will work rather than having a conversation about what does it mean to have a good life and what would you like to be doing with the time you have left, whether it is six months, two years, or five years. How much of it do you want spent in hospitals medicalizing things versus feeling good and doing the things you want to do? These are really hard conversations. Doctors struggle with them, as do patients. There's a lot we can do to have conversations early on before they are needed.[12]

Some people will say, "I want you to do everything possible for me. Don't give up," while other people will ask when they can stop treatment. The important thing is for you and your doctor to understand what you want and need.

THE TREATMENT PLANNING PROCESS

Unlike the paternalistic medicine once practiced in America, today's physicians seek a much more collaborative, patient-centered approach to treatment planning in which both the patient and family play a vital role. The goal is

> to develop an accurate, well-conceived treatment plan, using all available medical information appropriately while also considering the medical, social, and cultural needs and desires of the patient and family. A cancer treatment plan can be shared among the patient, family, and care team in order to facilitate care coordination and provide a roadmap to help patients navigate the path of cancer treatment.[13]

Not all goals are easily attained:

> There are numerous obstacles to achieving patient-centered cancer treatment planning in practice. Some of these challenges stem from the patient and include patients' lack of assertiveness, health literacy, and numeracy, and their emotional state and concurrent illnesses. Others are a result of physician limitations, such as a lack of time to

explain complex information and a lack of tools to facilitate treatment planning, as well as insensitivity to patients' informational, cultural, and emotional needs.[14]

There are other frequently cited reasons for inadequate participation in treatment planning:

The complexity of treatment options—each with its own set of potential risks and benefits—and the life-threatening nature of cancer and its emotional repercussions make it difficult for people with cancer to make decisions about their care. In addition, the fragmented nature of the cancer care system, involving multiple specialties, providers, and locations, also presents challenges that may impede coordinated care and the development of comprehensive treatment plans.[15]

If you wish to be an active participant in your treatment planning, there are a host of questions to which you will need answers. The American Cancer Society suggests starting with the basics:

- What type of cancer do I have? What is the stage or extent of my cancer?
- What is my outlook for the future (prognosis), as you see it?
- What treatment do you suggest and why?
- What is the goal of treatment—to cure or to control my symptoms?
- What are the possible risks or side effects of treatment?
- What are the pros and cons of the treatment you recommend?
- Are there other treatments for me to consider?
- How often will I need to come in for treatment or tests?
- How long will treatment last?
- What if I miss a treatment?
- What kind of changes will I need to make in my work, family life, and leisure time?
- How will we know whether the treatment is working?
- Why do I need blood tests, and how often will I need them?
- If other specialists take part in my care, who will be in charge of my treatment plan?
- What symptoms or problems should I report right away?
- If I do not feel sick, does that mean the treatment is not working?

- What are the chances that the cancer may come back (recur) with the treatment plans we have discussed?
- What can I do to be ready for treatment?
- Will I still be able to have children after treatment?
- Are there any special foods I should or should not eat?
- Can I drink alcoholic beverages?
- How much will treatment cost? Will my insurance pay for it?
- Should I think about entering a clinical trial?[16]

If you need more information, probe further:

- Is the recommended treatment driven by recognized guidelines or other protocols?
- Are there other treatment options available for my disease based upon its staging and grade, my age, and my personal health status?
- Are there unique aspects of my condition that make one option more appropriate than another?
- How arduous and lengthy will the recovery be after treatment?
- How will you know if treatment is successful?
- If the treatment is not successful, what treatment options will follow?
- How many times has the physician performed the recommended procedure?
- How urgent is the treatment, and why?
- How costly is the treatment (relative to value gained)?
- Does the physician whom you have selected to perform the treatment have any economic interest in your chosen treatment that may encumber his objectivity?
- What happens if I choose to do nothing?[17]

Once you have the answers to these questions, you are armed with a great deal of information about your disease, treatment options, and a recommended treatment plan.

Remember:

Pilots don't take off without a flight pattern, and architects don't break ground without a blueprint. Patients diagnosed with cancer are taking the journey of their life, literally, so the role of the cancer treatment plan in starting a conversation, in promoting comprehension and retention, in managing expectations and anxiety, and providing continuity across settings and episodes is so important.[18]

TOOLS TO HELP YOU

Treatment plans can take many forms but generally include comparable elements, including:

- all essential diagnostic and prognostic information;
- proposed methods of treatment, including sequencing/timing (all modalities);
- potential side effects or adverse consequence of treatment that must be monitored;
- adverse consequences from treatment that may appear at a later date;
- the designated roles and responsibilities for each member of the patient's care team;
- psychological, social, functional, economic, and spiritual support services as needed and desired; and
- palliative and/or end-of-life care planning as appropriate.[19]

The important thing is that you are completely informed of all your treatment options.

There are a variety of tools available online from such organizations as the American Cancer Society, National Cancer Institute, and American Society of Clinical Oncology (ASCO) that are designed to help you make informed decisions about your treatment plan:

> NCCS [National Coalition for Cancer Survivorship] offers the Cancer Survival Toolbox, a tool that helps patients diagnosed with cancer develop skills to help navigate their cancer treatment, including how to communicate, find information, make decisions, and negotiate and stand up for one's rights as a patient. In addition, ASCO publishes an advanced cancer communication guide that helps patients and their families understand their advanced cancer diagnosis, what options are available to them, and how to cope and locate support near the end of life. AHRQ provides a number of patient guides for

people with various types of cancer that help empower patients, including a list of questions patients should ask their providers.[20]

A LACK OF INFORMED CONSENT CAN LEAD TO POOR DECISIONS

Informed consent requires that a patient understand all the salient facts about a recommended treatment—from risks and benefits to available options. Ethicists and researchers agree that "Failure to obtain adequate informed consent compromises patient autonomy, places patient safety at risk, and legally may constitute negligence or battery."[21] Yet, there is a strong sentiment among researchers that, despite its importance, physicians often fail to obtain informed consent from their patients. One frequently cited reason for this omission is a lack of understanding by the patient regarding their physicians' recommendations.[22]

A prime example can be found by examining the data regarding women afflicted with stage 1 breast cancer. Unless there are other underlying issues, such as the presence of a BRCA mutation, these women have the option of selecting a lumpectomy followed by radiation versus a mastectomy. Though multiple research studies have confirmed the comparable effectiveness of either approach, "recent studies found that only half of early-stage breast cancer patients knew that patients treated with mastectomy and those treated with lumpectomy followed by radiation have equivalent survival outcomes, and only 11% of patients were able to answer three questions about breast reconstruction correctly."[23]

Sepucha provides an important perspective on stage 1 breast cancer:

> We really are seeing that the person who has to live with the consequences of these treatments should be the one figuring out what to do (or should play a very important role in figuring out what to do).
>
> In a situation like stage 1 breast cancer, we have good evidence, from over twenty years of randomized trials, that survival is the same whether you have a lumpectomy or a mastectomy. So it's not about survival.
>
> But these procedures are very different—and not just cosmetically. Keeping your breast comes with six weeks of radiation. It comes with a chance of reincision or multiple surgeries. It comes with the

need for a mammogram in six months—so there is some anxiety there. So different people may look at all of this and say, "You know what? I know I can keep my breast, but that's not my biggest driver—my biggest driver is getting back to work" or "Six weeks of radiation doesn't sound like a good thing" or "I'm really worried about side effects."

Not everyone is healed the same way. It might be different from what the doctor would choose. That can be difficult for the doctor. If they have a strong preference, they wonder why everyone else doesn't think the same way they do. But patients don't think the same way, and it's about giving patients a voice. [24]

It is not just breast cancer patients who suffer from a lack of comprehensive and objective information upon which to make treatment decisions. Sepucha, in discussing the outcomes of her research co-conducted with the University of Michigan, offered these powerful observations about the lack of truly informed consent and thus shared decision making:

What was striking was how little any of the patients knew. We looked at the kind of conversations people were having with their doctors. So we asked them if their doctor talked about the reasons to have the surgery or the reasons not to have the surgery, and did the doctor ask them what they wanted to do. Pretty consistently, across these different areas, we found that doctors were twice as likely to talk about the pros versus the cons, and only about half the time did doctors ask the patients what they wanted to do. So there are huge gaps in shared decision making. It is not something that is happening routinely across the country today. [25]

AN INDEPENDENT SOURCE OF TRUSTWORTHY INFORMATION

What you—and every cancer patient—should be seeking is trustworthy, unbiased information that represents a consensus of the best medical opinions regarding how to diagnose and treat your cancer. Such knowledge will raise your awareness of options and empower you to participate actively in your treatment.

That is why I am recommending a short side trip on your journey—a visit to the National Comprehensive Cancer Network's (NCCN) website, which is a repository of invaluable information for consumers, as well as physicians, and a "not-for-profit network of 25 of the world's leading cancer centers."[26] The primary mission of the NCCN is to develop and disseminate treatment guidelines, often referred to as "pathways," that represent "best practices" when managing various types of cancer.[27]

NCCN presents these pathways in detailed clinical terms for providers and then translates the information into language that is more easily understood by consumers. Far from being a superficial explanation, these patient guidelines can easily exceed one hundred pages in length for a single disease.

The list of NCCN "Guidelines for Patients" is constantly expanding. It currently includes some of the most commonly diagnosed cancers, including breast, colon, esophageal, non-small cell lung, ovarian, pancreatic, and prostate cancers and chronic myelogenous leukemia, melanoma, malignant pleural mesothelioma, and multiple myeloma, as well as caring for adolescents and young adults (AYA), and lung cancer screening.[28] All of this material can be viewed or downloaded at http://www.nccn.org/patients/guidelines/default.aspx.[29]

Once you have reviewed the guideline for your particular disease, you should have a far better understanding of:

- the definition of the disease,
- potential determinants of risk for the disease,
- possible indicators of the disease,
- primary methods of diagnosis,
- how a particular type of cancer is staged,
- advanced testing,
- treatment options—in general,
- how staging impacts treatment options, and
- side effects of different options.

There are factors that the guidelines likely won't address, including:

- the impact of a given treatment on your self-image,
- the level of geographic variation in recommended treatments,
- cost of recommended treatment,

- potential for conflicts of interest, and
- potential consequences of abdicating treatment.

There are numerous other trusted sources that patients can tap into for information. High on the list for any patient should be the Cochrane Collaboration, a British not-for-profit organization that provides information on the comparative effectiveness of various treatment options. It is a "loosely connected global alliance of 30,000 volunteer experts supported by 50 paid staff members."[30] The Cochrane staff is dispersed worldwide—including staffing an office at Johns Hopkins Hospital. Together, these individuals seek to analyze information and synthesize it into a systematic review that can be easily understood by patients as well as doctors. One major point of positive differentiation for the Cochrane Collaboration is "its meticulous attention to detail [and] . . . a reputation for incorruptibility in the face of pharmaceutical and medical device company inducements."[31]

Major cancer providers, such as the Mayo Clinic, Memorial Sloan Kettering, MD Anderson Cancer Center, and other NCI-designated facilities, often offer a wealth of patient-friendly information on their websites.

WHEN PHYSICIANS DEVIATE FROM CLINICAL GUIDELINES

Even when guidelines clearly exist, your physician may choose an alternate course of treatment. Do not assume that your physician is making a mistake by deviating from what you understand to be an established pathway. Rather than serving as absolute rules, pathways provide step-by-step treatment guidelines that have proven effective for the majority of patients with specific diagnoses. Nuances of your personal condition could dramatically change the protocols that are appropriate for you.

If your physician is taking a nonstandard care path, ask him or her why. Ask if he or she follows a particular set of evidenced-based pathways. Explain that you have reviewed the NCCN pathways, and it appears that you are receiving a different course of treatment than is standard for your disease. Your physician should be able to explain his or her decisions to you in clear and cogent terms.

If your physician seems defensive or balks at addressing your questions, ensure that you are framing your concerns in an objective fashion. If he or she still seems put off by your inquiry or suggests that you simply defer to his or her judgment, perhaps you should consider a second opinion before proceeding. We have more to say on that topic in chapter 7.

WHO IS IN CONTROL?

Despite your lack of medical training, you can nonetheless play an important role in determining your treatment. The question is whether you will step up to the plate and assume a degree of control for the management of your cancer.

Researchers seeking to understand the role of patients in decision making evaluated 10,939 decisions made by 5,383 patients with lung or colorectal cancer: "We asked patients to report their roles in decisions about surgery, radiation therapy, and/or chemotherapy to assess whether characteristics of the decision influenced patients' role in that decision. Of 10,939 decisions . . . 38.9% were patient controlled, 43.6% were shared, and 17.5% were physician controlled."[32]

What made the difference? The researchers responsible for this study concluded that the degree of control exerted by patients was a function of the level of evidence supporting the treatment recommendation:

> When there was good evidence to support a treatment, shared control was greatest; when evidence was uncertain, patient control was greatest; and when there was no evidence for or evidence against a treatment, physician control was greatest (overall p = .001). Decisions about treatments for metastatic cancers tended to be more physician controlled than other decisions (p = .001).[33]

If we return to our example of a woman with stage 1 breast cancer who can opt between lumpectomy and mastectomy, the research suggests, "Only about half the time did patients report that their doctor asked which treatment they wanted. In another analysis, only 60% of the time did patients and surgeons agree that both lumpectomy and mastectomy treatment options were discussed."[34]

COLLABORATIVE DECISION MAKING: FINDING THE RIGHT BALANCE

Patient-centered treatment plans require collaboration between you and your physician. This middle ground between deference and self-determination appears to be the best balancing point for many patients:

> Although most patients wanted to play an active role in decision making, they also sought the expert guidance of clinicians to ensure an optimal decision. Where clinicians seemed overly committed to relying on patient preference, and especially where they interpreted that to require withholding their own opinion, patients struggled with being confident in the correctness of their decisions.[35]

Remember: It is your body and your life! Cancer treatment is not about deference to a higher medical authority but rather a cooperative, informed, and shared decision-making process.

WHEN FEELINGS WIN OUT OVER FACTS

Patients sometimes choose procedures for which there is little to no scientific justification. One of the clearest examples can be seen in breast cancer patients who opt for contralateral mastectomies (in which both breasts are surgically removed) despite the complete lack of scientific evidence supporting such treatment for their particular disease:

> Contralateral prophylactic mastectomy (CPM) for patients with unilateral breast cancer is a glaring example of the need for greater clarity about the clinical logic of performing a more aggressive intervention to largely address patient reactions to the management plan.
>
> The rate of CPM for unilateral breast cancer increased from 39 to 207 per 1,000 mastectomies between 1998 and 2008. . . . The removal of the unaffected breast does not confer additional benefit with regard to distant disease-free survival in patients at average risk of a second primary breast cancer. . . . Patients should be encouraged to deliberate longer and to more directly consider the powerful cognitive and emotional reactions that may favor the most aggressive treatment approaches.[36]

As Sepucha observes, "The other thing that is happening now is that the pendulum may be swinging too far and women are saying, 'You know what? If you are going to take one breast off, why don't you just take both breasts off, and then I won't have to worry about this anymore?' If this is about anxiety, then we have better treatments for dealing with the anxiety than surgery."[37]

OTHER IMPORTANT FACTORS THAT CAN IMPACT YOUR TREATMENT

Before you can make an informed decision about the right treatment, there are a few additional things you should know—factors that may play into which path your physician recommends.

As noted, the most obvious factor influencing your physician's treatment recommendations may be his or her training. A surgeon may naturally gravitate toward surgical solutions, just as a radiation oncologist may see radiation as the preferred modality. The ideal situation is when representatives from the major disciplines involved in your treatment confer in a tumor board or case conference, weighing the pros and cons of various approaches before developing a treatment plan.

Another factor influencing your treatment may be where you happen to live. Believe it or not, it can be a major determinant of the type of treatment you receive. This radical discovery was first made by John Wennberg and Alan Gittelsohn, when, on a hunch, they examined the rates of tonsillectomies in two towns that were separated by mere miles. They discovered a radically different and unexplainable variation in the rates of tonsillectomies among the children in the towns.[38] The study was so disturbing to the status quo of medicine that it was rejected for publication by every major medical journal. It was finally published in the prestigious journal *Science*.[39]

As they continued their research over time, they discovered that medicine was rife with such geographic variation. Even today, four decades after the publication of their first article, such unexplainable variation exists. That means, for instance, that there can be a double-digit rate of variation in the use of mastectomies versus lumpectomies in the treatment of stage 1 breast cancer based purely on geography.

There is another even more disturbing factor that can influence the treatment you receive—financial conflicts of interest on the part of your doctor. Some physicians have an ownership interest in specific treatment modalities. An example would be the ownership of radiation therapy centers by urologists. By owning the equipment and being able to direct patients to their centers, urologists have reaped tremendous profits. The result has been double-digit growth in the use of radiation to treat patients with prostate cancer. Though radiation is an appropriate treatment modality for many prostate cancer patients, it is important that every patient is able to make an informed choice about treatment options without being unduly influenced by physicians who have an overt conflict of interest.[40]

This practice is perfectly legal. It becomes a concern, however, when such urologists consciously or subconsciously "push" this treatment option over other modalities that may be more appropriate for the patient. Hence, it is important to discern whether your physician has any financial interest in the interventions he or she is recommending that go beyond their customary professional fees for clinical services. Though your doctor is ethically obligated to disclose any conflicts of interest, in practice many physicians fail to do so.

If you doubt the role that economics plays in defining your treatment, consider this quote from a research study: "In a separate survey of oncologists, 58% said they considered revenue when making treatment recommendations. If a particular treatment would result in revenue loss, then most said they would choose to refer patients to a hospital (69%) or would prescribe an alternative medication (59%)."[41]

It's essential that you have complete confidence and trust in your oncologist as you embark on the journey ahead. If you have any concerns, address them now with the goal of leaving as many of your doubts behind as possible.

A FINAL ADMONITION

We began this chapter by talking about Stephen M.'s decision to take his foot off the accelerator and slow down. He needed to be deliberate about the decisions he was about to make. Lori agrees with him. If an oncologist with twenty-five years of experience suggests slowing down, shouldn't you?

We know it is not easy. There is tremendous momentum behind the need to make a treatment decision, as is captured in the following thought:

> A diagnosis of breast cancer and the sudden escalation of decisions trigger powerful emotional reactions from patients. Patients generally feel well at the time of diagnosis but suddenly confront a major health threat, a complicated decision context, and an arduous treatment course. Virtually all treatments that confer lifetime benefit are initiated in the first few months after diagnosis, and the decision-making process is generally compressed into the first few weeks. A sense of urgency in treatment planning is reinforced by the experiences of family and friends, by the powerful messages in the media, and by some clinicians who advise patients to initiate treatment quickly. Consequently, it is understandable that many patients want to do everything they can to leave this intense period of health threat, treatment decision-making, and treatment delivery behind— to move on with their lives with greater peace of mind. However, a consequence of this urge to leave it behind is the desire by many patients to quickly embrace all possible cancer treatments regardless of the level of benefit.[42]

Here's our best advice on how to proceed: Review patient-friendly versions of nationally published guidelines on the treatment of your type of cancer and then discuss what you have read with your doctor. If necessary, ask your doctor to fill in any gaps. Before proceeding with a decision about your treatment, you should be able to answer the following questions:

- Do I have a clear and unambiguous diagnosis?
- How do my diagnosis, stage, and my tumor's characteristics impact my prognosis?
- How will my performance status impact my ability to receive and benefit from treatment?
- Is my disease considered "curable" or "treatable"? What can be predicted about its progression?

- Based on my diagnosis, tumor characteristics, and performance status, is there a pathway that defines the sequence of treatments I should receive?
- Do I have a clear understanding of all my treatment options?
- Do I truly understand both the short-term and long-term adverse effects I could suffer as a direct result of my treatment(s)?
- Will I likely reach a point when the benefits of treatment are overshadowed by either my physical condition or the impact of treatment on my quality of life? If so, will my doctor tell me when that day arrives?

Then, with this information in hand, meditate, pray, or simply sit silently. Though it is difficult to quiet your mind in the face of relentless anxiety, it is the key to arriving at the right answers. Allow the information you have processed in your head to filter into your heart and your gut before making a decision. Given time, the answers will come.

Before concluding this chapter, Lori wants to offer two important points of caution:

- Beware of friends and family members who offer recommendations regarding your treatment based upon anecdotal accounts of acquaintances with your disease. Though well intentioned, they may be misinformed.
- If you feel paralyzed by an overwhelming amount of information coupled with the powerful emotional reaction that often accompanies a diagnosis of cancer, slow down and ask your care team for help. It's more important to make the right treatment decisions than to rush into decisions you may later regret.

6

UNDERSTANDING CLINICAL TRIALS

Clinical trials are a multistep process for testing the comparative effi-cacy (effectiveness) and safety of newly developed drugs and other ther-apies under investigation for use by physicians. Such trials can also be used to investigate new purposes for older drugs. For example, "Retrovir (zidovudine, also known as AZT) was first studied as an anti-cancer drug in the 1960s with disappointing results. Twenty years later, researchers discovered the drug could treat AIDS, and Food and Drug Administration approved the drug, manufactured by GlaxoSmithKline, for that purpose in 1987."[1]

Depending on the nature of your condition, your physician may suggest that you consider participation in such a trial. Clinical trials are most commonly associated with chemotherapy but also occur in other treatment modalities, such as surgery and radiation therapy. Currently, only approximately 3 percent of cancer patients in the United States are on clinical trials.[2] However, many experts believe that this number should be considerably higher due to the need to evaluate the relative effectiveness of different and emerging treatment methods.

Before deciding to participate in a trial, it is essential that your ex-pectations are appropriate. That means understanding the nature of clinical trials, as well as the benefits and risks you could experience.

A MULTIPHASED APPROACH TO CLINICAL TRIALS

The Food and Drug Administration (FDA) oversees all clinical trials. Before granting permission for the launch of a new trial, a pharmaceutical company must submit an investigational new drug (IND) application that describes the intended trial and provides evidence, from animal studies, that it appears safe to test the drug in humans. The IND must be reviewed and approved by both the FDA and a local institutional review board (IRB). Once approved, the drug proceeds through a number of distinct phases.

Phase 1 clinical trials are limited in size and can involve healthy subjects: "The goal here is to determine what the drug's most frequent side effects are and, often, how the drug is metabolized and excreted."[3] It is essential that you understand that "most phase I trials do not convey any therapeutic benefit and carry a risk of adverse effects. Studies reveal that many patients have limited understanding of the primary research aims, unrealistic expectations about benefits and risks, a questionable appreciation of their right to abstain or withdraw, and little knowledge about alternatives to phase I trial participation."[4] In other words, phase 1 is purely about safety. Assuming no overt problems surface in phase 1, the process continues.

Phase 2 begins to examine a drug's efficacy:

> This phase aims to obtain preliminary data on whether the drug works in people who have a certain disease or condition. For controlled trials, patients receiving the drug are compared with similar patients receiving a different treatment—usually an inactive substance (placebo), or a different drug. Safety continues to be evaluated, and short-term side effects are studied. Typically, the number of subjects in Phase 2 studies ranges from a few dozen to about 300.[5]

A very small number of drugs make it all the way through the pipeline to phase 3: "These studies gather more information about safety and effectiveness, studying different populations and different dosages and using the drug in combination with other drugs. The number of subjects usually ranges from several hundred to about 3,000 people."[6] Most of the studies offered to patients are phase 3 studies. Drugs that appear safe and effective at the end of phase 3 are formally submitted for approval via a new drug application (NDA) filed with the FDA. The

FDA seeks to review and rule on such applications within ten months of submission.

PRIMARY PURPOSE OF CLINICAL TRIALS

The primary purpose of a clinical trial is not to benefit you, as an individual patient, but rather to develop knowledge that affords the "greatest good for the greatest number." As such, you may not receive any direct benefit from your participation in a clinical trial other than the knowledge that you are involved in a process designed to help others in the future. In fact, you may have a 50 percent chance of not even receiving the investigational drug.

Patricia H. was given the option to participate in a clinical trial late in treatment. Though she knew the odds of it providing any meaningful remission were extremely small, she nonetheless enrolled because "I've gotten so much out of medical research. If I can give something back that helps in some way, I want to do that."[7] In an e-mail update to friends and family, Darrell described Patricia's options:

> The clinical trial would involve hospitalization for a period of at least 30–45 days, with intensive chemo at the start of that period to try to induce a remission. There is some risk of dying during that period due to infection—the chemo would destroy Patricia's bone marrow. Due to extensive precautions, the doctor said that risk is probably less than 10%, but it exists. If the treatment worked, it would have a 50% or better chance of producing a remission lasting from 1 to 2 years. The remission, if it happened, might well include improvement or elimination of the rheumatoid symptoms that have caused her so much pain and discomfort.
>
> The clinical trial consists of two groups: one group receiving the current standard of care treatment, the other (test) group receiving the trial drug, currently known as CPX351. It is a phase 3 trial, which means the trial drug has shown enough good results in phases 1 and 2 to merit continuing, and is approaching FDA approval. Patricia wouldn't get to choose which group she's in—that's randomly assigned by computer—but would be told which treatment she was getting. Again, the 50% success rate in producing a 1–2 year remission is for the current standard of care treatment; the hope and the early indications are that the trial drug may succeed at a higher rate.

Patricia asked me to tell all of you that she's taking this decision very seriously, with prayer and careful thought. On the one hand, the potential for positive outcomes from the clinical trial is appealing, as is the chance to advance medical knowledge and potentially help future patients. And, of course, who knows what other, better treatments might be found during that extra one or two years? On the other hand, going through a long hospitalization and intense treatment, with the very real possibility that it wouldn't bring about a remission, is daunting after all that she's already been through—she's confident that she's safe in God's arms, is tired, and has to decide if she has the emotional strength to face the difficulties of the clinical test path.

God's getting a few more tears to hold as I type this, but I'm so thankful that Patricia and I are not alone as she faces this tough decision. We have all of you—and that's an unspeakably precious gift—and we're both absolutely convinced that God is with us.

Grace and peace,
Darrell[8]

Some patients are fortunate enough to be involved in a study that yields positive results. Rarely does the drug under investigation prove to be a "silver bullet," but it can prove to slow the progression of a disease, thus affording the patient additional precious time with loved ones.

CRITERIA FOR PARTICIPATION

Clinical trials have strict criteria governing patients' participation in or exclusion from studies. These criteria can include demographics, health factors and performance assessments, location and stage of disease, and past or current treatment modalities being received by the patient.

Patients are often disappointed to learn that they are not candidates for a clinical trial. However, there are important reasons for inclusion or exclusion:

- These criteria help ensure the relative safety of patients participating in the trials.
- The criteria ensure that patients fit a profile congruent with the research objectives.

- The criteria help to eliminate confounding variables that may confuse the results of the trials.

Remember: The goal is to safely demonstrate the effectiveness of the treatment and also to ensure that the demonstrated efficacy is attributable to the therapy and not some other form of intervention that the patient is receiving: "Each clinical trial follows a set of rules called a protocol. A protocol describes inclusion and exclusion criteria; the schedule of tests, procedures, medications, and doses; and the length of the study."[9]

TYPES OF CLINICAL TRIALS

When seeking to determine the relative effectiveness and safety of an intervention, clinical trials may compare the intervention under investigation to an existing therapy or to a placebo, though the use of placebo is rare in cancer trials. The most rigorous of these studies are known as randomized controlled trials (RCT). In a randomized controlled trial, elaborate measures are taken to ensure that participants are randomly assigned to the different groups in which various interventions are being compared. The control group denotes those individuals receiving either a placebo or an existing therapy versus the intervention under study. The participants are unaware of their group designation and thus have no knowledge of whether they are receiving a therapeutically active therapy or a "sugar pill."

In a double-blind study, not only are the patients blinded as to their assigned group but so, too, are the researchers. Such a process eliminates any potential bias on the part of the researcher that can influence the study.

INVESTIGATORS AND FUNDERS

Clinical trials require four elements:

1. a sponsor who will fund the cost of the research;
2. a principal investigator (PI), who is responsible for the project;

3. approval of an IRB; and
4. FDA approval to proceed.

It is important that you understand the issue of sponsorship:

> Clinical trials are sponsored by government agencies such as the
> National Institutes of Health (NIH), including the National Cancer
> Institute (NCI), pharmaceutical companies, individual doctors,
> health care centers such as health maintenance organizations
> (HMOs), and organizations that develop medical devices or equip-
> ment. Clinical trials can take place in hospitals, universities, doctors'
> offices, or community clinics. [10]

Historically, the majority of clinical trials were conducted by academic organizations; one example of such a group is the Eastern Cooperative Oncology Group (ECOG):

> The Eastern Cooperative Oncology Group (ECOG) was established
> in 1955 as one of the first cooperative groups launched to perform
> multi-center cancer clinical trials. A cooperative group is a large net-
> work of researchers, physicians, and health care professionals at pub-
> lic and private institutions across the country who are members of
> the group. Funded primarily by the National Cancer Institute (NCI),
> ECOG has evolved from a five member consortium of institutions on
> the East Coast to one of the largest clinical cancer research organiza-
> tions in the U.S. with almost 6,000 physicians, nurses, pharmacists,
> statisticians, and clinical research associates (CRAs) from the U.S.,
> Canada, and South Africa. Institutional members include univer-
> sities, medical centers, Community Clinical Oncology Programs
> (CCOPs), and Cooperative Group Outreach Programs (CGOPs).
> These institutions work toward the common goal of controlling, ef-
> fectively treating, and ultimately curing cancer. Research results are
> provided to the world-wide medical community through scientific
> publications and professional meetings.
>
> Currently, ECOG has more than 90 active clinical trials in all
> types of adult malignancies. Annual accrual is 6,000 patients, with
> more than 20,000 patients in follow-up. [11]

Academic organizations and such groups as ECOG, generally speaking, have no inherent bias relative to demonstrating the efficacy and
safety of a drug. Pharmaceutical companies and medical device manu-

facturers, on the other hand, can stand to reap significant profits from drugs that successfully emerge from the clinical trials process.

In recent years, a great deal of pharmaceutical research has shifted away from academic organizations and aligned cooperatives to contract research organizations (CROs). A CRO is a for-profit, independent company that provides clinical research for a fee at the behest of its pharmaceutical clients. Though the PI on a study can reside within a major academic organization, the CRO exerts tremendous control over the research process and may determine which resulting information from the study is within the purview of the PI to see.

Research sponsored by pharmaceutical companies, conducted under the auspices of CROs, is being heavily scrutinized due to concerns about the validity of some of the research. Much of the research is conducted in foreign countries, where the investigational protocols are far more lax than the standards demanded by NCI-sponsored trials. If you wish to learn more about this issue, consider reading *Bad Pharma* by Ben Goldacre.

NUMBER OF PATIENTS PARTICIPATING IN CLINICAL TRIALS

The number of patients enrolled in clinical trials is a small fraction of the total population of adult cancer patients:

> Despite the promise offered by clinical trials, less than 5% of adults with cancer enroll in them. This low level of participation slows progress in the development of new, more effective therapies. By contrast, more than 60% of children with cancer receive treatment through a clinical trial. Approximately three-quarters of children with cancer survive long-term, compared with half of adults. The increased survival rate for children can be directly linked to the enrollment of patients in cancer clinical trials over many years whose experience led to better treatments and better outcomes.[12]

However, clinical trial enrollment at NCI-designated cancer centers is much higher than in community settings. In fact, a key determinant of eligibility for designation as an NCI cancer center is the enrollment of at least 15 percent of all patients in clinical trials. For those patients wanting the assurance that their case is being given appropriate consideration for participation in a trial, an NCI center may be most appropriate.

QUESTIONS TO ASK BEFORE CONSIDERING A CLINICAL TRIAL

The NIH offers a list of questions that candidates for clinical trials may wish to ask their physicians. The answers can provide invaluable information in helping you determine whether a specific clinical trial is right for you:

- What is being studied?
- Why do researchers believe the intervention being tested might be effective? Why might it not be effective? Has it been tested before?
- What are the possible interventions that I might receive during the trial?
- How will it be determined which interventions I receive (for example, by chance)?
- Who will know which intervention I receive during the trial? Will I know? Will members of the research team know?
- How do the possible risks, side effects, and benefits of this trial compare with those of my current treatment?
- What will I have to do?
- What tests and procedures are involved?
- How often will I have to visit the hospital or clinic?
- Will hospitalization be required?
- How long will the study last?
- Who will pay for my participation?
- Will I be reimbursed for other expenses?
- What type of long-term follow-up care is part of this trial?
- If I benefit from the intervention, will I be allowed to continue receiving it after the trial ends?
- Will results of the study be provided to me?
- Who will oversee my medical care while I am in the trial?
- What are my options if I am injured during the study?[13]

ADDITIONAL CONSIDERATIONS BEFORE AGREEING TO PARTICIPATE

It is important to understand the potential adverse effects of participating in the trials—not only in terms of potential long-term consequences but also regarding the possible diminution of your quality of life. Remember, a clinical trial is rarely a reprieve from your prognosis. In rare instances, it brings new hope of slowing the progression of the disease by offering a superior treatment. In all instances, it furthers our understanding of what does and does not contribute to effective cancer treatment.

It is also important to understand the financial ramifications of participating in trials. Some expenses may not be covered by your insurance, including certain imaging studies that are conducted throughout the trial period and travel to and from the facility where you will receive care. You should speak with the financial counselor associated with your cancer center to understand your potential financial liability.

THE LUCKY FEW

Some patients *do* experience positive outcomes from novel therapies tested in clinical trials. Susan Gubar, a humanities professor at the University of Indiana and a frequent contributor to the *New York Times*, is one example. The following excerpt from the June 26, 2014, issue of the *New York Times* tells of her experiences as an ovarian cancer patient in a recent clinical trial:

> When I signed up for this clinical trial of a medication never before used on human beings, I was informed that Phase 1 studies do not extend life. They are designed to test dosage and toxicity. Since August 2012, however, the pills, as yet unnamed, have been keeping my recurrent ovarian cancer at bay.
>
> Like many people, I am concerned that only a small percentage of trials results in protocols more effective than what is already available. And the prices of newly marketed therapies seem outrageous. Some new drugs blight the end of life with their miserable side effects or cause secondary cancers. Even when catastrophic conse-

quences do not occur, hideously ingenious malignancies can and often do become resistant to sophisticated interventions.

Given all these apprehensions, imagine my growing astonishment as the experimental drug in my trial continues to keep me in remission.[14]

FINDING A TRIAL

The best way to find a trial is through your physician. He or she can determine if your disease warrants potential participation in a trial, whether an appropriate trial exists, and if you meet the eligibility criteria. Your doctor can also ensure that you are fully informed before providing consent to participate.

If your physician is unable to help you find an appropriate trial, we have listed a number of resources for learning about potential trials at the end of this book.

7

THE IMPORTANCE OF GETTING A SECOND OPINION

You are facing some of the most difficult and important decisions of your life related to your diagnosis, prognosis, and available treatment options—decisions that should be driven primarily by you, your family, and your care team. Decisions of such magnitude, almost by definition, invite a second opinion.

The National Cancer Institute (NCI) provides excellent guidance on how to obtain a second opinion:

> You can do this by asking another specialist to review all of the materials related to your case. The doctor who gives the second opinion can confirm or suggest modifications to your doctor's proposed treatment plan, provide reassurance that you have explored all of your options, and answer any questions you may have.
>
> Getting a second opinion is done frequently, and most physicians welcome another doctor's views. However, some people find it uncomfortable to request a second opinion. When discussing this issue with your doctor, it may be helpful to express satisfaction with your doctor's decision and care and to mention that you want your decision about treatment to be as thoroughly informed as possible.
>
> You may also wish to bring a family member along for support when asking for a second opinion. It is best to involve your doctor in the process of getting a second opinion, because your doctor will need to make your medical records (such as your test results and x-rays) available to the specialist who is giving the second opinion.

Some health care plans require a second opinion, particularly if a doctor recommends surgery. Other health care plans will pay for a second opinion if the patient requests it. If your plan does not cover a second opinion, you can still obtain one if you are willing to cover the cost.[1]

As you contemplate whether to seek a second opinion, consider that the research reveals that "overwhelmingly, patients find second opinions helpful."[2]

Many patients are so confident in their physicians that they see no reason to corroborate their doctors' findings or recommendations. Dana B. is a perfect example: "I knew the credentials of all of the people I was seeing. I had an initial consult with all of them and felt comfortable in the way they handled and approached my situation. I felt that they were all very personable and compassionate. So I went with it and moved forward. I trusted that they knew best."

WHERE TO SEEK A SECOND OPINION

Here you must examine what is practical versus what is ideal for your particular circumstances. It could be argued that the best place to receive a second opinion is from a physician who treats a large number of patients with your diagnosis and experiences positive outcomes relative to the prognosis for this particular disease. Such physicians often practice within major NCI-designated cancer centers.

There are a number of practical hurdles to surmount, however, including:

- obtaining consent from the specialist (and his or her facility) to see you,
- the costs associated with traveling to a facility that may be far from home, and
- the emotional challenges of being in a "strange" facility far from home and loved ones.

If you have a rare or advanced disease, you will probably want to receive an opinion from the best and brightest experts you can find. If, however, you are dealing with a more commonly treated form of cancer with well-established pathways, you might seek a second opinion from a specialist within your community.

If you seek a second opinion within your community, there are a few guidelines to consider:

- Request a second opinion from a physician who is unaligned with your current medical provider.
- You may, in fact, want to consider a physician who practices at a different medical facility.
- Be sure you understand the credentials and qualifications of the physician rendering the second opinion. We strongly encourage you to review the criteria for evaluating doctors found in chapter 3.

WHAT A SECOND OPINION COULD REVEAL

You stand to gain a great deal by obtaining a second opinion—beginning with the reassurance that your physician's diagnosis, prognosis, and treatment recommendations are accurate and appropriate. That is most frequently the case.

Shelley W. found that a second opinion simply bolstered her confidence in her physician's findings and recommendations: "We got a second opinion on my films as well as an oncology opinion. I again got referrals from my nurse. I wanted to see someone from a different institution just to see if they agreed, and they did."[3]

However, there are instances where changes to the diagnosis and prognosis are warranted and alternative treatment recommendations are made. Though these cases are statistically small in number, they have profound ramifications to the patients:

> . . . according to a study that reviewed the biopsy slides of 6,171 patients referred to Johns Hopkins Medical Institutions for cancer treatments, 86 patients had diagnoses that were significantly wrong and would have led to unnecessary or inappropriate treatment.
>
> The rate of error was 1.4 percent, which is low, but not insignificant. At Johns Hopkins alone, it would be equal to about one cancer patient a week with a wrong diagnosis, and across the country could add up to a conservative estimate of 30,000 mistakes a year.

For 20 patients, a second opinion changed a malignant diagnosis to a benign one. In five other cases, a growth reported to be benign was later found to be malignant, and in six cases one type of cancer had been mistaken for a different type. . . .

In a 1998 study at the University of Texas Southwestern Medical Center in Dallas, a review of ovarian, uterine, cervical and vulvar biopsies found major errors in 2 percent of the cases, leading doctors to cancel six operations and five chemotherapy treatments. And a 1997 review of patients who went to the University of Texas M. D. Anderson Cancer Center for second opinions of their brain and spinal cord biopsies found major errors in 8.8 percent of cases.[4]

According to an article appearing in *Cancer World*, "Another study of 148 women who went to the University of Michigan Breast Care Center for a second consultation following a mammogram found that 7% had more cancer in the same breast, or an undiagnosed tumour [*sic*] in the other breast."[5]

A second opinion could also bring to light new information about your treatment options. This information falls into one of four categories: (1) advising against a recommended procedure because of a substantive change in diagnosis, as seen in the previously mentioned research; (2) offering new treatment interventions based on cutting-edge research and knowledge not available to your physician; (3) providing stronger admonitions regarding potential side effects, including long-term adverse consequences of treatment; and (4) modifying the treatment plan to reflect a change in diagnosis from a benign to a malignant tumor.

WHO SEEKS SECOND OPINIONS?

Although many people might benefit from a second opinion, a far smaller group of patients actually seek them. In fact, we know from the research that "patients seeking second medical opinions are not representative of the whole patient group. In attempting to characterize these patients, Tattersall et al. found they generally had higher education levels, worked in managerial or professional positions, and were more likely to be female than the whole population presenting to cancer outpatient clinics."[6]

People's motivations for seeking a second opinion vary. A study of fifty-two patients with advanced cancer revealed that

> Seventeen of the fifty-two (33%) patients had sought a SMO [second medical opinion], most commonly prompted by concerns around communication with their first doctor, the extreme and desperate nature of their medical condition and the need for reassurance. Most (94%) patients found the SMO helpful, with satisfaction related to improved communication and reassurance.[7]

WHY DO PATIENTS CHOOSE NOT TO SEEK SECOND OPINIONS?

Patients are often afraid of offending their physicians—someone whom they will likely count on to win their battle with cancer. Patients believe that a request for a second opinion is akin to questioning the judgment and clinical knowledge of their doctors. However, you can enjoy a good, trusting relationship with your doctor and still request a second opinion. A second opinion should never be viewed as a vote of no confidence in your existing medical team.

HOW PHYSICIANS VIEW SECOND OPINIONS

In general, research seems to suggest that "Physicians regarded SMO patients as having greater information needs (84%), greater psychosocial needs (58%) and requiring more of the physician's time and energy (77%) than other patients."[8]

Here is what Lori has to say about patients' requests for second opinions:

> When a patient raises the issue of a second opinion, I don't take it personally. Rather, I welcome it! Having another set of eyes on the patient and their clinical data serves the patient's best interests. There are times when another opinion may slightly alter the treatment plan. Remember: There is not usually just one way to approach treatment. A second opinion, at the very least, offers reassurance and

peace of mind to the patient, family, and physician—which is worth a great deal.

Though strongly endorsing second opinions, Lori adds a note of caution:

> Two things concern me about second opinions, and both represent potential dangers to patients. First, the patient needs to understand that a second opinion may take time and even delay therapy. Usually, this is not a critical issue, but when I feel timing is crucial, I sometimes suggest we take initial steps to plan the patient's treatment while he or she pursues another opinion.
>
> Second, there are those rare physicians who offer opinions based more upon self-interests than the medical needs of the patient. Granted, these doctors are the outliers and thus represent a small percentage of the medical profession. Even so, it is important when seeking a second opinion that the recommendations be consistent with mainstream, evidence-based pathways.
>
> I remember one patient who had the courage to ask her oncologist why he was recommending chemotherapy that was in conflict with other physicians' opinions and not part of a national guideline. He became enraged by her challenge to his authority and gave her no legitimate reason. If not for her questioning, she would have received an inappropriate and toxic chemotherapy.

A SECOND OPINION DOES NOT NECESSITATE RECEIVING ACTIVE TREATMENT OUT OF TOWN

Though patients may opt to receive a second opinion from a major cancer center, that does not necessitate that they receive treatment at that facility. Often major cancer centers refer the patient back to their local specialist armed with observations and recommendations regarding their treatment plan. In other cases, a major referral center may perform the initial phase of treatment, such as the surgical removal of a tumor, but recommend that ongoing treatment be performed by local providers.

NOT ALL EXPERIENCES ARE POSITIVE

Darrell H. relates an experience he and his wife, Patricia, had when seeking a second opinion from a cancer expert a few hours' drive from home:

> At one point we went up to Omaha to see a specialist. Patricia went in to see her while I waited in the lobby taking care of Meghan [our daughter]. Patricia came out looking just devastated. She said that the doctor told her that she had eight years maximum to live, and that includes the two years that have already passed working on the diagnosis. It made me aware that, though we want the truth, the way it gets communicated by a physician can make a big difference. It was really rough. After Patricia passed the eight-year mark, we'd refer back to this time and say, "Maybe the doctor didn't know every-thing."[9]

COORDINATION OF CARE IS AS IMPORTANT AS WHERE THE CARE IS DELIVERED

The crucial issue is not simply who provides the care but the need for tight coordination and communication between all of the physicians involved in your case. Academic medical centers are somewhat notori-ous for failing to communicate adequately with their referral sources, which can be deleterious to patient care. Though you should not have to be the conduit for the smooth flow of information between doctors, you will likely be required to do so. The value of a second opinion far outweighs the additional effort.

II

During Active Treatment

8

THE EMOTIONAL ROLLER COASTER OF CANCER

For many cancer patients, the emotional roller coaster that began at the time of diagnosis may continue well into treatment. It's hard to imagine not feeling distressed when one faces a life-altering disease. In fact, emotional distress is so common that it is recognized as the "sixth vital sign in cancer care, calling for systematic allocation of supportive resources."[1]

Emotional distress often goes unaddressed during the early stages of diagnosis and treatment—a time when, ironically, intervention may be most beneficial. Dana B. expressed regret that the offer of psychological assistance didn't arrive until she was done with treatment: "At the end of my treatment, there was a referral card for a psychologist. I felt like it was a little late in the game. If anything was missing, it was probably the encouragement to seek psychological healing. It would be helpful for someone to say, 'You are going to experience a lot of these feelings. You may want to hook up with someone who specializes in this area.'"[2]

For patients like Dana, emotional distress manifests in many ways. Patients may feel sad, afraid, hopeless, anxious, discouraged, and even exhausted. It is the intensity, frequency, and duration of these feelings that determine whether they are a normal, emotional reaction to cancer or something more significant.

WHEN DISTRESS CROSSES THE LINE AND BECOMES MORE SERIOUS

It's important to bear in mind that there is no sharp line in the sand separating "normal" distress from more debilitating levels of anxiety, depression, and posttraumatic stress. However, according to the American Cancer Society, there are warning signs that may indicate the need for some level of intervention, including:

- Feeling overwhelmed to the point of panic
- Being overcome by a sense of dread
- Feeling so sad that you think you cannot go through treatment
- Being unusually irritable and angry
- Feeling unable to cope with pain, tiredness, and nausea
- Poor concentration, "fuzzy thinking," and sudden memory problems
- Having a very hard time making decisions—even about little things
- Feeling hopeless—wondering if there is any point in going on
- Thoughts about cancer and/or death all the time
- Trouble getting to sleep or early waking (getting less than 4 hours of sleep a night)
- Trouble eating (a decrease in appetite, or no appetite) for a few weeks
- Family conflicts and issues that seem impossible to resolve
- Questioning your faith and religious beliefs that once gave you comfort
- Feeling worthless and useless[3]

YOU ARE NOT ALONE

If your anxiety or depression has reached clinically significant levels, you are not alone. We know from extensive research that a meaningful percentage of cancer patients will be so affected—though many patients with distress go undiagnosed. How large a percentage is a topic of great debate: "Variability in reported prevalence rates . . . ranged from 0% to 46% for depression and 1% to 49% for anxiety."[4]

Two major studies, however, suggest that approximately 20 to 45 percent of patients experience clinically significant anxiety, depression, or both. One of the studies included more than 4,000 patients treated at a major cancer center. The researchers found that 18.7 percent of patients had "significant depressive symptoms, and 24% had significant anxiety symptoms."[5] The second study examined more than 10,000 patients over a five-year period and concluded that "19.0% of patients showed clinical levels of anxiety and another 22.6% had subclinical symptoms. Further, 12.9% of patients reported clinical symptoms of depression and an additional 16.5% described subclinical symptoms."[6]

Though there may be ongoing debate about the level of clinically significant emotional distress among cancer patients, there is little debate as to when such distress is most likely to occur: "It is generally agreed that anxiety and depression are highest at the time of diagnosis and decrease over time, with levels of anxiety and depression typically returning to a level comparable to the general population around two years post-diagnosis."[7] It is important to note that some patients' first experience with clinically significant anxiety or depression occurs post-treatment. Some patients experience strong fears of recurrence without the comfort conveyed by ongoing treatment.

ANXIETY VERSUS DEPRESSION

As you may have noted from the research findings, there has been a tendency to categorize patients' distress as indicative of either anxiety or depression. This artificial dichotomy often leads to the use of selective medicines for treating a single disorder. It now appears that a number of distressed patients have symptoms of *both* anxiety and depression and should be treated accordingly.

CERTAIN PATIENTS ARE MORE LIKELY TO EXPERIENCE DISTRESS

Though distress may be a universal human reaction to a cancer diagnosis, we know that some people are more affected than others:

- Women experience greater rates of anxiety and depression than men. Based on their type of cancer, these rates may be two to three times as great as those found in men.[8]
- Age can play a significant role, with younger patients experiencing higher levels of distress (anxiety and depression).[9]
- A prior history of psychological distress is a major risk factor for rekindling anxiety or depression in cancer patients.
- Education, social status, levels of physical activity, and other factors also determine one's vulnerability to emotional distress.

WHO IS MONITORING MY DISTRESS LEVELS?

Despite the prevalence of distress, don't count on your physician to address your mental health or well-being. The reality is that physicians do an inadequate job of identifying and addressing the psychological needs of their cancer patients. That is not our opinion but rather empirical fact supported by research: "In recorded discussions between oncologists and patients less than a third of consultations contain discussions of emotional concerns such as distress or depression."[10] As one physician told me, "I wait for the patient to bring it up. I don't initiate conversations about their feelings."

In one survey of oncologists, only 14 percent reported screening for distress with an evidence-based tool, and one-third reported that they didn't routinely screen for distress at all. Because doctors are often focused on physical symptoms and treatment, studies have found emotional and psychological issues may be overlooked or discounted. Patients, for their part, may be too embarrassed or reluctant to report their concerns. And while large cancer centers have the resources and staff to screen for distress and provide help, community hospitals and oncology practices—where about 85 percent of cancer patients in the United States get their care—often don't have the time or funding.[11]

Such neglect is not due to the lack of clinical tools used in diagnosing clinically significant distress. Though researchers constantly debate the merits of various psychological tests, the truth is that there is a myriad of tools that can provide quick and powerful insights into your mental health or well-being. Clinicians have access to such tests as the Beck Depression Inventory (BDI) or the Hospital Anxiety and Depression

Score (HADS), which require nothing more than a pen or pencil and a few minutes of your time to complete.

An even more basic "test" of distress involves the "Distress Thermometer" developed by the NCCN (see figure 8.1). You can download the "Distress Thermometer" from the NCCN website and complete it before visiting with your doctor.

If you are feeling unduly anxious or depressed, it is important that you talk to your physician about it. Ask him or her if there is a social worker in the office or other mental health professional with whom you may speak. If not, you may want to ask for a referral. In many communities, there are cancer support organizations that address this gap in

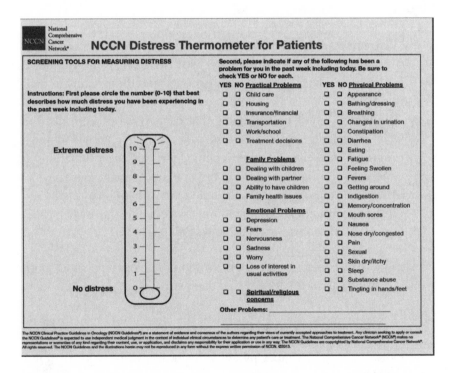

Figure 8.1. **NCCN Distress Thermometer for Patients Reproduced with permission from the NCCN Clinical Practice Guidelines in Oncology (NCCN Guidelines) for Distress Management V.2.2014. 0 2014 National Comprehensive Cancer Network, Inc. All rights reserved. The NCCN Guidelines and illustrations herein may not be reproduced in any form for any purpose without the express written permission of the NCCN. To view the most recent and complete version of the NCCN Guidelines, go online to http://www.nccn.org/.**

care. If you are suffering, it is important that you seek out empathic
providers who can help you manage the emotional roller-coaster ride.

THE NEGATIVE EFFECTS OF DISTRESS

There are two excellent reasons for addressing your distress: (1) There
is no reason to suffer undue anguish if it can be remedied; and (2) there
are very real physical consequences to impaired mental health or well-
being. Even if you believe in a stoic approach to suffering, such an
approach could negatively impact your physical well-being.

Once again, it is helpful to look at what can be gleaned from the
research (even though the research is a bit difficult to decipher from a
lay perspective). We now know that:

- "Untreated, distress may have long-term detrimental consequences on patients' compliance with treatment, survival, desire
  for hastened death, and on both patients' and their relatives' quality of life."[12]
- "While it may not be surprising that cancer can prompt distress,
  what is striking is that distress can affect a patient's physical
  progress. Not only can such feelings interfere with the ability to
  cope with the rigors of cancer therapy, experts say, but they can
  lessen one's motivation to complete treatment. They can also
  interfere with the body's immune system and have a negative
  impact on the course of the disease."[13]

Though still controversial, there is mounting evidence that one's
level of distress can ultimately impact one's survival:

- "A recent meta-analysis [a statistically significant, structured re-
  view] of 25 observational studies showed a 39% higher all-cause
  mortality rate in cancer patients diagnosed with major or minor
  depression."[14]
- "A recent prospective study of psychosocial issues and breast cancer survival found a significantly increased risk of death by 5 years
  from all causes in women with high scores for depression and
  helplessness/hopelessness."[15]

- "On the other hand, a well known study of newly diagnosed cancer patients by Cassileth et al. found that 'the inherent biology of the disease [cancer] alone determines the prognosis.' Others have subsequently confirmed this finding."[16]

Moira Mulhern is a clinical psychologist and founder of Turning Point—a not-for-profit organization committed to addressing the psychosocial and spiritual needs of patients. Now part of the University of Kansas's NCI-designated cancer center, Turning Point treats approximately 10,000 patients per year. When asked about the potential impact that psychosocial interventions might have on prognosis, Dr. Mulhern offered this observation:

> For sixteen or seventeen years, I ran a group of stage 4 cancer patients. Many of the patients lived well beyond their prognosis—in fact, they lived eight, ten, fifteen years with no obvious explanation as to why they were still alive. Was it a result of the things we were doing to improve their lives? Was it exercising? Was it self-calming and acceptance of their condition? I know that the majority of them sought to live every day fully. Is that what kept them alive? I don't know.[17]

What we do know for certain is that emotional distress takes a toll. How heavy a toll is a topic of debate, but there is little argument over the need for better identification and treatment of clinically significant symptoms of anxiety, depression, and other related disorders in cancer patients.

TAKING ONE'S OWN PULSE

The best way to measure your levels of distress is by working in partnership with health care professionals who are trained to administer certain tests—beginning with the "Distress Thermometer." If this option is not readily available, you can use self-administered tests that provide important insight into whether further testing may be advisable. The two conditions you may wish to monitor are depression and anxiety, which, as previously noted, often coexist.

Numerous psychological tests are available on the Internet. Because these tests vary dramatically in their scientific foundations and hence value, you need to look for tests that:

- have proven validity (a good indication of validity is that they are recommended by a trusted resource);
- are easy to administer;
- are self-scoring; and
- provide a quick, easily understood evaluation of the level of your distress.

Two sites that you may wish to explore are:

- http://www.am-i-depressed.com/zung-depression-scale.html and
- http://www.authentichappiness.com, where you will find a wide array of tests measuring well-being, including a depression test (CES-D).

The American Cancer Society also publishes a self-assessment questionnaire on their website designed to help reveal whether patients could benefit from professional support.

NEW MANDATE

In recognition of the importance of addressing emotional distress, new standards are being adopted for evaluation and referral of cancer patients: "Starting in 2015, the Commission on Cancer, which accredits centers that treat about 70% of all new cancers diagnosed in the U.S., will require providers to meet a new standard to evaluate patients for distress and refer them to programs for help."[18] We hope that this new standard will help reduce the level of undiagnosed distress endured by a sizable percentage of cancer patients.

COPING 101

Although cancer may be the most daunting challenge you have faced to date, there undoubtedly have been other difficult periods during your lifetime. You probably discovered a variety of methods for coping with these stressful times that could prove quite effective in improving your well-being during cancer treatment and survivorship.

Some of these strategies involve other people, including family, close friends, and clergy. Other strategies are solitary endeavors. Whatever brings you peace, comfort, meaning, or joy should be considered. Here are some of the myriad ways that cancer patients reduce their stress levels and improve well-being:

- **Physical Activity.** Exercise, as is discussed in greater detail in chapter 10, has been shown to have a profound effect on stress and well-being. Consider new forms of exercise, such as yoga, that may be easier to manage while undergoing treatment.
- **Quiet and Contemplation.** This could take the form of meditation, prayer, guided imagery, or similar practices.
- **Journaling.** The simple act of writing about your experiences and feelings can be profoundly cathartic.
- **Practicing Gratitude.** Gratitude exercises for the many "gifts" that you still enjoy and enrich your life have been demonstrated to have a powerful effect on well-being.
- **Maintaining Normalcy.** Seek to maintain those aspects of your life that make it feel "normal" and hold onto as much of your daily routine as possible.
- **Support Groups.** Experiment with support groups to determine if they are helpful for you.

Many communities are fortunate enough to have dedicated cancer resource centers that provide well-being services. Ask your physician or nurse about the types of services available in your community. You can also search the Internet. It is best if you can find services offered by a not-for-profit, community organization whose mission is to improve patients' well-being.

WHEN SOME ADDITIONAL HELP IS NEEDED

When your existing methods of coping fail to bring adequate relief from distress, take comfort in knowing that numerous additional interventions are available, including supportive therapies (i.e., talk therapies), medicinal therapies, physical activity, and positive psychology interventions.[19]

Supportive Therapies (Talk Therapies)

Patients who seek supportive or talk therapy will likely receive care from a psychologist, psychiatric social worker, counselor, or similarly trained professional. These mental health professionals may employ a variety of techniques to help patients reconceptualize their distress, including cognitive behavioral therapy.

Some patients may be more comfortable seeking counsel from members of the clergy who are trained in pastoral counseling:

> Pastoral services are important because finding out you have cancer can lead to a crisis of faith or belief. Some people may question the purpose of their life or wonder why God "gave" them cancer. Others may feel that God is punishing them or that God has left them. Still others may use their religious and spiritual resources as a means to cope with their illness and help them sort through these kinds of questions.[20]

Medical Therapies

If medical therapies are indicated, your physician will either prescribe drugs designed to mediate your anxiety and/or depression or refer you to a psychiatrist or psychiatric nurse practitioner. While antianxiety drugs generally take effect immediately, the benefits from antidepressants may not be evident for two to four weeks.

It is important for you to understand the benefits, limitations, risks, and side effects of any medication prescribed to you. You should also ensure that new medications do not interact with any current medications and that there are no dietary restrictions associated with taking the new medications.

Physical Activity

As previously indicated, physical activity is among the most powerful interventions known for improving well-being. It is discussed extensively in chapter 10. For now, suffice it to say that an approved exercise plan can make a tremendous difference in your overall mental health and ability to endure the rigors of treatment.

Positive Psychology Interventions

The final group of interventions is derived from the emerging field of positive psychology. Whereas psychology traditionally has focused on what is wrong with patients, positive psychology seeks to build on what is *right*. Its focus is on enhancing well-being and mitigating the damaging effects of distress. Though it has been occasionally derided for being focused on *happiness*, positive psychology is a scientifically rigorous discipline that has yielded important findings about how to enhance meaning, fulfillment, joy, and vigor in our lives.

Among the most researched positive psychology interventions is mindfulness, a form of meditation that is quickly learned and easily practiced. Though it may have little to no impact on the physical course of a patient's disease, it can improve quality of life, acceptance of one's condition, and the ability to smooth out the bumps in the long journey through cancer.

Other forms of positive psychology interventions commonly used with cancer patients include:

- resilience training,
- gratitude exercises, and
- music therapy.

For additional information regarding these and other therapies, visit these websites:

- http://www.health.harvard.edu/newsletter_article/Positive_psychology_in_practice
- http://www.authentichappiness.org

THE TRANSFORMATIVE BENEFITS OF DISTRESS

"I'm one of those people that will say, 'My cancer was a gift.'"[21]
—Melissa Etheridge

Some cancer patients are able to transform distress into an opportunity for significant personal growth and change. When this happens, distress, rather than engendering anxiety and depression, exerts a positive effect on patients' lives.

> Many interventions have been developed to help women cope with both the physical and psychological negative effects of diagnosis and treatment. However, there is evidence that extremely significant events, such as cancer, can impact a person's self-concept, relationships, and values, which can mean a reorganization of life's priorities as the person attempts to achieve a better and healthier life. Dealing with cancer can lead to positive changes, which may emerge spontaneously or be elicited through the suitable psychological intervention.[22]

As Bill E. puts it, "There ain't nothing I can't do! There's nothing I can't accomplish. Right now, I have the mindset that I'm going to live forever. I really do! Nothing is going to stop me from moving forward."[23]

YOUR TAKE-AWAY MESSAGE

People's emotional reactions to cancer are as varied as their personalities. Even so, the preponderance of anxiety, depression, and other conditions that negatively impact patient well-being are well documented. If you are feeling a moderate to high level of distress, it is important to discuss this issue with your doctor. Depending on the significance of your symptoms, you may benefit from a variety of treatments, ranging from physical activity to meditation to medication.

You can learn to manage your distress and benefit significantly in the process. As Dr. Mulhern observes, "After all of these years of working with patients, I keep finding that the most important thing is the ability to manage anxiety, to self-calm. It allows you to think, make better decisions, feel more at peace, and enjoy a higher quality of life in the midst of it all."[24]

9

METHODS TO MINIMIZE SIDE EFFECTS

Side effects vary greatly based upon the nature of one's disease and the treatment being received. For example, patients diagnosed with head and neck cancers often experience a wide range of side effects related to their treatments, as was the case with Ali H.:

> My doctors tried to prepare me for what to expect. They told me that I might have a rash, dizziness, severe nausea, fevers alternating with chills. I would not be able to go out in the sun. I would lose my saliva glands as well as the lymph glands in my neck. My immune system would go down. They said that I would probably lose my hair and that my eyelashes might curl up under my eyelids and have to be removed professionally. My fingernails might start to crack and split.
>
> They also told me that I might never be able to taste again. That was very tough for me; I was a food and beverage person. I was passionate about it. I was a certified sommelier. I did wine tasting and wine training. I loved doing it! I realized that I was going to lose my ability to do something that I am passionate about. I would have to find something new to feel passionate about. That was a difficult issue for me psychologically.
>
> They painted a pretty ugly picture. I would rather have someone tell me the worst possible scenario. Once I accept it, anything less becomes great.
>
> The side effects did not hit me physically until almost the fifth week of treatment. Then I understood what they were talking about. Once they began, it was difficult. [1]

These are just some of the side effects that Ali experienced following treatment for his head and neck cancer. Side effects refer to the unintended consequences of treatment. They represent a profound issue in cancer treatment for patients who undergo debilitating surgeries, ingest highly toxic medical cocktails, and are irradiated until they fear that they will glow in the dark. It's no wonder that there's some level of collateral damage to their bodies.

Ali—and other cancer patients—will quickly tell you that the better you understand the likelihood of developing such side effects and the degree to which they can be managed, the more likely you are to minimize their negative impact on your life.

THE UBIQUITOUS NATURE OF FATIGUE

The most commonly experienced side effect of cancer treatment is fatigue or exhaustion, which is sometimes referred to as *cancer-related fatigue* (CRF). The overall prevalence of CRF is estimated to approach 50 percent, with higher prevalence in selective types of cancer, including breast cancer, lymphoma, and pancreatic cancer.[2]

Fatigue arises whether patients are receiving radiation, chemotherapy, or other modalities. When it strikes, "patients with cancer become too tired to participate fully in the roles and activities that make life meaningful; the most important impact of fatigue may be in the realm of quality of life (QOL)."[3] In fact, CRF is viewed as among the most debilitating of all side effects:

> Among all symptoms that tend to affect cancer patients in particular—e.g., pain, sleep disturbances, lack of appetite, or nausea—those of CRF are perceived as most distressing. CRF markedly impairs the quality of life and the physical performance ability of many of the affected patients. Multiple prospective studies have shown an association of the manifestations of CRF with shorter survival and increased mortality. CRF can arise at any point in the course of the disease: It may be an early symptom even before the cancer is diagnosed, or it may arise during the treatment, long after the treatment is over, or when the disease recurs or progresses.[4]

Despite its prevalence, physicians often fail to ask their patients about fatigue. As a result, many patients fail to receive any form of treatment that could be beneficial in alleviating their CRF.[5]

MANAGING CANCER-RELATED FATIGUE

Despite our lack of understanding about many of the mechanisms underlying CRF, physicians are nonetheless able to offer various types of treatments that could be quite helpful. The first step, of course, is ensuring that you and your physician are actively aware of the problem as it arises rather than waiting for it to become a chronic condition.

The methods used to treat CRF range from counseling to exercise to medications. Often, these interventions are combined for optimal effectiveness. The main goals of treatment are:

- alleviating any factors that may be worsening the patient's CRF,
- offering individualized help so that the patient can cope with the symptoms and stresses of CRF, [and]
- activating the patient's strengths and resources.[6]

It is also recommended that your caregiver participate in the treatment of CRF. Because caregivers often mirror symptoms of the patient and are likely to experience fatigue as well, including them in elements of the treatment program, such as exercise, may be preventative. Furthermore, it enhances empathy for the patient's struggle with fatigue.

A LAUNDRY LIST OF ADDITIONAL SIDE EFFECTS

Fatigue is the most commonly experienced side effect, but there are hundreds more, many of which are treatment specific. Because of the infinite number of treatment combinations, it is virtually impossible to predict all the ways side effects might manifest. Before you begin any form of cancer therapy, whether surgery, chemotherapy, or radiation, your physician should review a comprehensive list of side effects as part of the informed consent process.

If you want additional information on the potential unintended consequences of treatment, there are a few excellent sources of information available on the web. Two of the most trustworthy sites that provide detailed information are:

- National Cancer Institute (NCI), http://www.cancer.gov/cancertopics/coping/physicaleffects
- American Cancer Society (ACS), http://www.cancer.org/treatment/treatmentsandsideeffects/physicalsideeffects/physical-side-effects-landing

What follows is a brief summary of some of the most commonly experienced side effects associated with chemotherapy, radiation, and surgery and what can be done to relieve or remedy them. It is important to keep in mind that, as a general rule, the greater the intensity of treatment, the higher the probability of side effects.

COMMON SIDE EFFECTS FROM CHEMOTHERAPY

Dana B. remembers when she first started chemotherapy:

> I was all gung-ho. Let's go for it! Let's get this cancer out of me! Then I had my very first treatment of Adriamycin and Cytoxan, which is pretty brutal. The first one was a huge shock to my body. I thought, "I'll just go back to work," but I was walking around like a person out of my head. Finally, I just said that I had to go home. I can't do this!
>
> I remember calling my mom, crying, saying, "I don't know if I can do this!" I have a strong mom, so she said, "Yes, you can, and you will," which was helpful. I had sixteen treatments—four of the Doxorubicin [Adriamycin] and twelve of Taxol. The AC [Adriamycin Cytoxan] was not fun. It was every two weeks. After four or five days, I felt pretty good. The Taxol, weekly, was not nearly as toxic feeling, so I managed that pretty well. I had a good schedule. I'd go Thursday, go back to work on Friday, then have a pretty crummy weekend but be able to go back to work on Monday, so I missed very little work due to side effects from chemo.[7]

After reading Dana's story, it should come as no surprise that one of the first chemotherapy agents, known as *nitrogen mustard*, was derived from a chemical weapon used during World War I. This historical fact lends some insight into the toxicity of some chemotherapeutic agents. Not only are they capable of killing cancer cells, but they also wreak havoc on your system in the process. Common side effects associated with chemotherapeutic agents include:

- **Nausea and Vomiting.** Until the development of powerful drugs to control nausea and vomiting, these debilitating symptoms often accompanied certain forms of chemotherapy. Patients undergoing treatment with platinum-based chemotherapeutic agents, such as Cisplatin, often had to receive treatment for dehydration due to vomiting. Anti-emetics, such as Ondansetron, among others, now provide significant—though not total—relief.
- **Hair Loss.** Historically, chemotherapy was often associated with hair loss. Many of the traditional chemotherapy agents do produce this effect, which is almost always temporary in nature, with hair returning within a few months of treatment. More modern, targeted therapies rarely have this effect.
- **Cognitive Impairment and Fatigue.** These symptoms led to the term "chemo-brain," or "chemo-fog," referring to the confusion, memory changes, lack of energy, and related symptoms that often accompany chemotherapy.
- **Sepsis.** One of the most serious side effects of chemotherapy is sepsis, a potentially life-threatening, systemic infection brought about by low white blood counts that must be dealt with immediately. Signs of potential sepsis include a fever above 101° following chemotherapy, shaking, chills, rapid heart rate (above one hundred beats per minute), and more rapid respirations.
- **Changes in Complete Blood Count (CBC).** Chemotherapy can result in changes to your blood count. Patients may experience lowered red blood cells, causing anemia; lowered white blood cells, increasing the risk of infection; and lowered platelets, leading to difficulty with blood clotting. There may also be changes in blood chemistry, such as potassium, magnesium, and creatinine levels, which require close monitoring.

In addition to these side effects, patients can experience a variety of additional issues, including:

- diminished appetite;

- changes in bowel habits, including diarrhea and constipation;
- aches and pains in muscles, stomach, or jaw;
- difficulty with balance and walking;
- some loss of hearing;
- neuropathy; and
- sores in the mouth.

Fortunately, many of these symptoms are transient.

COMMON SIDE EFFECTS FROM RADIATION

Radiation is a powerful form of energy capable of destroying cancer cells. It can be delivered through external methods using a machine known as a *linear accelerator* or internally via radioactive implants or injections. Although advances in radiation therapy have allowed for much more precise targeting of the energy, some level of collateral damage to surrounding tissue is inevitable. This exposure of healthy tissue to radiation can produce a variety of side effects that generally occur within the area being targeted by radiation:

- **Skin.** External radiation must pass through the skin before reaching its intended target. In the process, the skin receives varying doses of radiation. The level of radiation absorbed determines whether the skin is slightly reddened, significantly irritated, or burned. When burns occur, they must be carefully managed to avoid infection.
- **Digestive Tract.** Certain parts of the body have an enhanced sensitivity to radiation, including the gastrointestinal (GI) tract. Significant irritation can occur when there is exposure to the esophagus, stomach, colon, rectum, and other parts of the digestive system. The irritation can manifest as nausea, vomiting, abdominal cramping, or diarrhea.
- **Major Organs.** As radiation passes through the tumor, it may also pass through crucial organs or other structures, such as the heart or spinal cord. Radiation oncologists go to great lengths to minimize such exposure, but sometimes it is inevitable. The con-

sequences of such exposure can be minor or major and immediate or delayed.

- **Breathing.** Radiation can have a powerful effect on the lungs. If a patient's lung function is already compromised due to preexisting conditions (such as asthma or chronic obstructive pulmonary disease [COPD]), radiation has the potential to worsen their problems.
- **Brain.** Radiation to the brain can result in a variety of complications, including overall cognitive impairment and changes in balance. Whenever possible, radiation oncologists attempt to limit exposure to the tumor site within the brain. However, when there are multiple tumors, as often occurs when certain cancers metastasize, "whole brain" radiation may be required.
- **Head and Neck.** Radiation to this area may cause short- or long-term changes to taste, saliva production, dental health, and swallowing.

In addition to enumerating these side effects, the NCI provides advice to patients regarding other issues they can experience based on the area receiving radiation. For more information, refer to http://www.cancer.gov/cancertopics/coping/physicaleffects/radiation-side-effects.

Bill E.'s radiation to his head and neck predictably damaged his salivary glands, leading to a perpetual dry mouth: "I have dry mouth. I take a bottle of water with me wherever I go, whether it is a meeting or a ball." Though it's annoying, he considers it a small price to pay for surviving a difficult bout with cancer.[8]

Your radiation oncologist can provide you and your caregiver with tailored information regarding the side effects that can accompany your specific treatment and what can be done to manage them.

COMMON SIDE EFFECTS FROM SURGERY

As is true with any invasive procedure, cancer surgery carries risks. These risks can be related to anesthesia, incision and excision, and wound healing. Surgical side effects may or may not be avoidable, including:

- **Postoperative Infections.** Great progress has been made in reducing the rate of postoperative infections in recent years. Such infections are generally managed effectively with antibiotic therapy but can be very problematic for patients whose immune systems are compromised either from underlying disease or from certain forms of treatment.
- **Lymphedema.** When lymph nodes are surgically removed, patients can experience swelling and other symptoms in that area of the body. This condition occurs frequently with breast cancer patients who have undergone lymph node removal and radiation. Therapy can help patients learn to manage the symptoms of lymphedema, with varying degrees of effectiveness.
- **Cosmetic Issues.** Surgery can significantly change the appearance of one's body, which can be particularly problematic for patients undergoing breast surgery, surgery to the head and neck, and surgery resulting in ileostomies or colostomies (which necessitate that urine or stool drain into an external bag). Often one or more reconstructive surgeries are required to restore some degree of normalcy to one's appearance. It should be noted that surgical cosmesis (the cosmetic result following surgery) may be a function of surgical technique, experience, and competency.
- **Digestive Issues.** Removal of portions of the digestive system, as occurs in numerous types of GI cancers, can have a profound impact on digestion and appetite.
- **Sexual Function.** Sexual function can be directly affected by surgery, as is frequently the case for patients undergoing radical prostatectomies or removal of the ovaries. It may also be compromised by changes to body image, hormone levels, and other factors resulting from various types of surgery.
- **Neurological and Cognitive Issues.** Neurosurgery, whether to the brain or spine, can lead to a profound array of side effects, ranging from subtle changes in cognition to impaired mobility.

Some consequences of surgery may be due to surgical error. Errors run the gamut from failure to excise a tumor to damaging sensitive structures, such as the spinal cord. The consequences can be minor and transient or debilitating and ultimately fatal. Your best protection against such errors is to have a highly experienced surgeon who regularly performs your procedure operating in a well-regarded facility.

GOING THROUGH HELL TO HAVE A CHANCE AT LIFE

Some treatments can only be described as draconian and bring with them potent side effects that are not merely uncomfortable but life threatening. When Diane C. was diagnosed with acute myeloid leukemia, her doctors gave her a 20 percent chance of living—and that was only if she underwent a bone marrow transplant (BMT). Here's how Diane described the experience: "I was in the hospital for thirty days for induction (chemotherapy). It hits you like a ton of bricks. That was the toughest part of my whole treatment—having my immune system trashed in the hope of killing the cancer. If you live through it, you will be in good enough shape to have the transplant. I had five bad infections during this period. I nearly died."[9]

Fortunately, Diane survived. Today, seven years after being told that she had such a small chance of surviving, she is vibrantly alive: "I'm a poster child. I'm 100 percent. I have no sign of disease. When I go in for a checkup, they bring in the residents and even patients to show that people survive it."

WHEN TO TALK WITH YOUR DOCTOR

Before undergoing any form of treatment, you should have a crystal-clear understanding of the potential side effects that you may experience as a result of such treatment. Because some of these side effects can exert a powerful and lasting impact on your quality of life, it is important to keep the goals of your treatment in mind. If the intent is curative, then one's ability to accept and tolerate certain adverse effects may be increased. If, however, the intent is to provide symptom relief without the hope of cure, one has to weigh the adverse, unintended consequences of treatment against the anticipated benefits.

Every patient has a different "list" of the side effects he or she is willing to endure for a predicted outcome. The patient's age, medical condition, outside support, and inherent personal values also shape this list. In order for a patient to weigh the risks and benefits of treatment, they must be fully informed by their physician as to the goals of treatment as well as the anticipated side effects. Only then can a patient determine if the trade-offs between treatment and potential quality of life are appropriate for them.

TAKING A LONG-TERM PERSPECTIVE ON SIDE EFFECTS

Many side effects are experienced by patients within hours, days, or weeks of undergoing a specific type of treatment. Others, however, may not appear for months, years, or even decades after treatment has ceased. Therefore, it is essential that you understand not merely the immediate risks and discomforts of treatment but also the long-term sequelae (after-effects) of some treatments.

One of the most glaring examples of the delayed effects of treatment is apparent in survivors of certain types of childhood cancer. One study published by the American Society of Clinical Oncology in 2014 looked at the incidence of breast cancer (by age fifty) in 1,230 female survivors of childhood cancer. All participants had received radiation therapy to the chest. The study authors concluded that "The entire cohort had a 22-fold increased risk of breast cancer."[10] They also found that the women who developed breast cancer did so earlier in life, with a median age of thirty-nine when diagnosed.

Another long-term problem is infertility. Many chemotherapeutic agents, as well as some types of radiation, induce early menopause. If appropriately advised, some women can have multiple options for dealing with this consequential side effect, the most effective of which is to have their eggs harvested and frozen for later implantation. Recent research suggests that some breast cancer patients may also benefit from injections of a drug known as Goserelin or Zoladex, though additional studies need to be done to confirm this finding.[11]

BEING PREPARED IS HALF THE BATTLE

Assuming you proceed with treatment, one of the best ways to manage side effects is to be prepared. It's important to know in advance how to manage potential problems following treatment. Advance preparation may make the burden of side effects more manageable.

10

MAKE NUTRITION AND EXERCISE PART OF YOUR TREATMENT PLAN

My doctors told me that my treatment would cause me to have pain, and they said it would be tough to deal with. I would not be able to eat, so I would need to have a tube put into my stomach to provide liquid nutrition for several weeks. When the doctors said I might not be able to eat or drink due to treatment, I thought, "OK, the tube is my backup plan. What do I have to lose?" I had the tube put in before treatment started.

Treatment made everything taste bad. Things tasted bitter. I had trained my mouth to taste subtle nuances between wines, so I had a heightened sense of taste and felt the change more acutely. For a couple of weeks, I could not swallow anything—not even water.

I will say that the tube added another layer of pain to an already-difficult situation, but when I got to the point where I could not eat or drink, I was grateful I had done it. No one wants to have a tube in his or her body, but you are not dealing with a normal situation. You have to be prepared to do what it takes.[1]

Ali H. had learned "to do what it takes" at a very early age. When he was eighteen, the political situation in his native country of Iran became dangerously unstable. His father, who served as a general in the shah's army, feared for Ali's safety, and so he helped arrange for Ali to travel to America on a student visa. Shortly after arriving, Ali watched as the situation in Iran deteriorated—leading ultimately to the 1978 hostage crisis in Iran. It was then that he knew he would not be able to return. He would never see his parents again.

When Ali was diagnosed with cancer, he said the moment reminded him of when he first heard about the hostage crisis and had the emotion-filled realization about his parents. It would take courage and determination to move forward and deal with the cancer. He believed he had to maintain a positive attitude while enduring the hardship of cancer treatment.

When he started treatment, Ali weighed 192 pounds. When he finished, he weighed 157. It was not easy, but Ali got through it. Although he can no longer distinguish the subtle differences in wines, he now speaks of pursuing a new passion—teaching at the university level.

ABCS OF CANCER NUTRITION

When you are well, ensuring that your body gets the appropriate levels of nutrition and exercise takes only a modicum of work. However, when you have cancer, the challenge becomes far greater. It also becomes all the more important. Proper nutrition and appropriate exercise can make a tremendous difference in your ability to manage your disease and treatment as well as provide the benefit of a higher quality of life.

Cancer and its treatment may significantly affect your appetite and thus nutritional status. That is not surprising when you consider the assault on your system wrought by the disease coupled with the after-effects of chemotherapy, surgery, and radiation.

Chemotherapy and radiation can alter your sense of taste and smell. Fortunately, these are usually temporary phenomena. So, too, is the nausea and vomiting that can accompany treatment. Other common problems that limit appetite include mouth sores associated with treatment, difficult and painful swallowing, impaired digestion, and a host of other issues—all of which constitute a recipe for no appetite. As if that were not enough, add constipation induced by pain medications, stress-related anorexia, and the consequential effects of certain surgeries, and it is easy to understand how patients can lose vast amounts of weight.

Though virtually all cancer patients can benefit from a nutritional assessment, it is *essential* for those patients who have cancers known to place them at high risk of malnutrition. Top among such cancers are head and neck cancers and cancers of the digestive tract.

As part of their nutritional advice to patients, the National Cancer Institute (NCI) highlights problems associated with surgery to the head and neck:

- Surgery to the head and neck may cause problems with:

  - Chewing
  - Swallowing
  - Tasting or smelling food
  - Making saliva
  - Seeing

- Surgery that affects the esophagus, stomach, or intestines may keep these organs from working as they should to digest food and absorb nutrients.

All of these can affect the patient's ability to eat normally. Emotional stress about the surgery itself also may affect appetite.[2]

The problem with compromised nutrition is not merely the weight loss. Failure to obtain properly balanced nutrition leads to protein and vitamin deficiencies accompanied by weakness and difficulty healing, which can also exacerbate underlying cancer-related fatigue. A vicious cycle then ensues in which one grows progressively weaker and less able to cope with the rigors of treatment. Without proper nutrition, our bodies are less able to heal and are more prone to infection.

Poor nutrition can result despite our efforts to eat properly. Some cancers and treatments alter the body's ability to metabolize foods in a normal way. What may be an appropriate level of nutrition under normal conditions can suddenly prove inadequate—causing you to lose weight despite eating normally.

SCREENING AND ASSESSMENT

The first step toward ensuring a proper level of nutrition is a screening and assessment by your doctor as part of your diagnostic workup. He or she may begin with a short series of questions, including:

- What changes have occurred in your weight over the past twelve months? Is it continuing to change?
- Have there been changes in your diet, either in the type of food you eat or the amount?
- Are you experiencing side effects of treatment or other issues related to your disease that affect your ability to eat?
- Are you experiencing cancer-related fatigue?

Once these answers are in hand, your doctor will conduct a physical examination that includes checking your overall health, weight, muscle mass, and level of body fat. He or she will also use blood tests to measure the levels of protein and essential minerals in your body. Your physician may repeat this process often throughout your active treatment.[3] If one is available, a nutritionist can also participate in this process.

CHANGES IN WEIGHT AS A SYMPTOM OF DISEASE

Some cancer patients initially present with unexplained weight loss as a first sign of cancer. Cancer is a predator that competes with normal cells for nutrition within the body. Thus the cancer gets fed while your body is deprived of the nutrients it needs.

INTEGRATING A NUTRITIONAL PLAN INTO YOUR OVERALL TREATMENT PLAN

If your doctor determines that you are at risk of malnutrition, he or she may recommend nutritional therapy. In such cases, you will work with other members of the medical team, including nurses and dieticians. As a first step, the team will recommend modifications to your diet while continuing to monitor your weight.

In some cases supplemental nutrition may be recommended. For head and neck cancer patients, doctors could advise proactively implementing more aggressive methods for ensuring proper nutrition, including a feeding tube, as was the case with Ali. Prior to treatment, patients often resist this recommendation because they are feeling relatively well and may even need to lose weight. Only after they have endured difficult surgery, radiation, or chemotherapy do they realize the need for such support. It is far better to begin such support early.

If you think that Ali's case is the exception, here's what Bill E. said about the treatment for his head and neck cancer: "When I started chemotherapy, I was completely out of it. I just gave up. I was losing my balance and falling. With the radiation, I couldn't eat. I went from 220 pounds down to 170. I'm a big man, and suddenly I was thin, clothes weren't fitting, and I was cold all the time."[4]

PLANNING AHEAD

One of the most important things you can do is to anticipate potential nutritional issues and take steps in advance to help minimize problems. Perhaps the easiest and most basic way to add nutritional value to your diet is through liquid supplements, such as Boost, Ensure, or Carnation Instant Breakfast, all of which essentially offer a nutritious meal in a drink.

When it comes to nutrition, the American Cancer Society recommends that you "talk to your treatment team about the things that worry you. Many people have few or no side effects that keep them from eating. Even if you have side effects, they may be mild, and you may be able to manage them with drugs or simple diet changes. Most side effects go away after cancer treatment ends."[5]

The American Cancer Society also provides some practical suggestions about how to be prepared:

- Stock your pantry and freezer with your favorite foods so you won't need to shop as often. Include foods you know you can eat even when you are sick.
- Cook in advance, and freeze foods in meal-sized portions.
- Talk to your friends or family members about ways they can help with shopping and cooking, or ask a friend or family member to take over those jobs for you.
- Talk to your doctor, nurse, or a registered dietitian about any concerns you have about eating well. They can help you manage side effects like constipation or nausea.

For more information on coping, see the "To learn more" section and/or call your American Cancer Society at 1-800-227-2345.[6]

WHEN ADDITIONAL SUPPORT IS NEEDED

Sometimes patients are unable to take food by mouth due either to weakness or other physical conditions. In such cases, supplemental nutrition can be provided via several different routes—including enteral nutrition and parenteral nutrition:

> *Enteral nutrition* is giving the patient nutrients in liquid form (formula) through a tube that is placed into the stomach or small intestine. The following types of feeding tubes may be used:
>
> - A nasogastric tube is inserted through the nose and down the throat into the stomach or small intestine. This kind of tube is used when enteral nutrition is only needed for a few weeks.
> - A gastrostomy tube [or PEG] is inserted into the stomach or a jejunostomy tube is inserted into the small intestine through an opening made on the outside of the abdomen. This kind of tube is usually used for long-term enteral feeding or for patients who cannot use a tube in the nose and throat. . . .
>
> If enteral nutrition is to be part of the patient's care after leaving the hospital, the patient and caregiver will be trained to do the nutrition support care at home.[7]

Parenteral nutrition is administered intravenously:

> Parenteral nutrition is used when the patient cannot take food by mouth or by enteral feeding. Parenteral feeding does not use the stomach or intestines to digest food. Nutrients are given to the patient directly into the blood, through a catheter (thin tube) inserted into a vein. These nutrients include proteins, fats, vitamins, and minerals.
>
> Parenteral nutrition is used only in patients who need nutrition support for five days or more.[8]

THE BENEFITS OF PROPER NUTRITION

It is not easy to adhere to a diet when one feels acutely ill, nor is it pleasant to have a tube inserted into one's body for supplemental nutrition. The benefits, however, far outweigh the temporary assault to one's quality of life.

The NCI reminds us not only that "healthy eating habits and good nutrition can help patients deal with the effects of cancer and its treatment" but also that "some cancer treatments work better when the patient is well nourished and gets enough calories and protein in the diet. Patients who are well nourished may have a better prognosis (chance of recovery) and quality of life."[9]

The NCI delineates a number of specific benefits of nutritional therapy. It can:

- Prevent or treat nutrition problems, including preventing muscle and bone loss.
- Decrease side effects of cancer treatment and problems that affect nutrition.
- Keep up the patient's strength and energy.
- Help the immune system fight infection.
- Help the body recover and heal.
- Keep up or improve the patient's quality of life.[10]

FOOD-DRUG INTERACTIONS

Cancer patients must also be mindful of how the drugs they are receiving for treatment may interact with certain foods. Not only can these interactions change the relative effectiveness of the drugs, but dangerous side effects can also result. The following are some common examples:

- Grapefruit juice can intensify the effects of Targretin (Bexarotene).
- Alcohol, when combined with Folex or Rheumatrex (Methotrexate), can result in liver damage.
- The effectiveness of Mithracin (Picamycin) can be diminished by calcium and Vitamin D.

- Any type of food can limit the effectiveness of Temodar (Temozolomide).[11]

Your nutritional plan should clearly identify such potential interactions so they can be scrupulously avoided. Your medical team should also be aware of any herbal or complementary medicines that you are taking to ensure that there are no potential food-drug interactions (e.g., many patients take antioxidants, which can interfere with the effectiveness of their treatments).

ADDITIONAL ADVICE ON NUTRITION

There are plenty of web-based resources that give guidance on nutrition and how to manage side effects, including:

- National Cancer Institute's "Nutrition in Cancer Care (PDQ)," http://www.cancer.gov/cancertopics/pdq/supportivecare/nutrition/Patient/page1/AllPages, and
- American Cancer Society's "Nutrition for the Person with Cancer during Treatment: A Guide for Patients and Families," http://www.cancer.org/acs/groups/cid/documents/webcontent/002903-pdf.pdf.

THE IMPORTANCE OF EXERCISE

Exercise can have a profound impact on your ability to manage the journey through cancer. In fact, it is among the most important things you can do to improve your health, lower your risk of depression and anxiety, better tolerate treatment, enhance your well-being, and enjoy a better quality of life. "Physical activity . . . helps you maintain muscle mass, strength, stamina, and bone strength. It can help reduce depression, stress, fatigue, nausea, and constipation. It can also improve your appetite."[12]

Lori and I are extremely strong proponents of exercise. We know that it is a difficult habit for some patients to establish, particularly if they have been sedentary, are experiencing cancer-related fatigue, or are depressed. Yet when you consider the evidence supporting the benefits of exercise for cancer patients, it seems to be an essential part of most patients' treatment plan.

You do not have to take our word on this issue. A great deal of effort is going into research that examines the effects of exercise on cancer patients. To date, that research has yielded some important findings:

> The benefits of exercise are well documented in a number of cancers . . . namely in areas such as fatigue and physical functioning, both of which directly influence quality of life. While survival is the ultimate outcome measure, with an estimated 12 million cancer survivors and growing in the United States, the importance of improving quality of life has grown exponentially.
>
> The evidence linking physical activity with improved quality of life in those undergoing active treatment and those who have completed it "is incredibly strong," said Dr. Rachel Ballard-Barbash of NCI's Division of Cancer Control and Population Sciences. . . .
>
> Two of the primary goals of exercise . . . are improved body image and body composition. In the case of the former, many cancer patients undergo extensive surgery or receive treatments that can alter their physical appearance and radically alter feelings about things such as sexual attractiveness, said Dr. [Kathryn] Schmitz [of the University of Pennsylvania's Abramson Cancer Center]. "There's good evidence in the literature that physical activity can improve body image, and that may be one mechanism through which exercise can improve quality of life," she explained. . . .
>
> The guidelines also make note of the suggestive evidence—but by no means definitive evidence—in breast and colorectal cancer that regular exercise after treatment improves progression-free and overall survival. As the data continue to emerge in this area, a prescription for exercise could be "an adjunct to curative care." . . . But [researcher] Dr. Courneya acknowledged that the jury is still out on survival, calling the data "exciting" but "still experimental."[13]

> Early studies of exercise in patients with cancer indicated that exercise could increase functional capacity during chemotherapy, improve marrow recovery and decrease complications during peripheral blood stem cell transplantation, and decrease fatigue and other symptoms during radiation therapy and chemotherapy.[14]

PREVENTIVE BENEFITS OF EXERCISE

One of the most important emerging findings from research on exercise is its potent effect in preventing a number of different types of cancer. One key finding is the clear linkage between obesity, sedentary lifestyles, and the development of colon and breast cancer—a problem that appears to be reduced by exercise. Here are the facts:

> More than two dozen studies have shown that women who exercise have a 30 percent to 40 percent lower risk of breast cancer than their sedentary peers. The female hormone estrogen seems to play a key role. Women with high estrogen levels in their blood have increased risk for breast cancer. Since exercise lowers blood estrogen, it helps lower a woman's breast cancer risk. Exercise also reduces other cancer growth factors such as insulin.
>
> Even older women need to be concerned about estrogen, because after menopause the hormone is produced by fat cells. Women who exercise have less fat and therefore produce less estrogen. With more than 150,000 new breast cancer cases reported in the United States each year, preventing cancer through exercise is one of the best ways a woman can take charge of her health. . . .
>
> Exercise plays a dramatic role in preventing cancer of the colon and rectum. Nearly 150,000 Americans are diagnosed with colorectal cancer each year, and nearly 50,000 die from the disease. Encouragingly, more than three dozen studies show exercisers reduce their risk of colon cancer by 20 percent or more compared to sedentary people, and the benefits are seen in both men and women, although the effect is greater in men. Changes in digestive acids and other substances also occur with exercise, and these changes are believed to provide some protection from colon cancer. Decreases in body fat, insulin and other growth factors also may contribute to exercisers' lower colon cancer risk. Current research is also uncovering new ways in which physical activity cuts cancer risk—from reducing chronic inflammation to improving DNA repair.[15]

Exercise prevents far more than cancer. It can greatly reduce your likelihood of developing numerous chronic conditions, such as diabetes, high blood pressure, and other diseases that reduce your overall performance status. Remember that the two greatest determinants of your prognosis are the characteristics of your tumor coupled with your performance status.

Before you run out to the nearest gym, talk to your doctor.

INTEGRATING AN EXERCISE PLAN INTO YOUR OVERALL TREATMENT PLAN

Just as you worked with your team to develop a nutritional plan, you may benefit by having a medically approved exercise plan. Begin by talking with your medical team about the type and intensity of exercise in which to engage. Your physician may also recommend a consultation with exercise physiologists, physical therapists, and other professionals who possess specialized training and can provide you with a personalized exercise program. Prior to making recommendations, these professionals will consider such factors as whether there should be limitations on exercise based on your diagnosis and treatment, as well as how your general health and functional status might affect your exercise regimen.

The goal is to maximize the benefit you receive from exercise while minimizing the risk: "Specific risks of exercise training by cancer site should be understood by fitness professionals, such as elevated fracture risk among breast or prostate cancer survivors who have undergone certain types of hormonal therapy and lymphedema risk more commonly seen among breast and urogynecologic cancer survivors."[16]

The NCI cautions, "In men who have undergone androgen-deprivation therapy for prostate cancer, for example, trainers need to be aware of fracture risk and adjust the exercises accordingly. And many women with breast cancer will have had surgery that can [impair the functioning of] the shoulder, so the guidelines encourage the use of exercises to stabilize and strengthen the surrounding muscles."[17]

THIRTY MINUTES, THREE TO FIVE TIMES PER WEEK

If medically appropriate, your goal should be to engage in moderate aerobic exercise for a minimum of thirty minutes, three to five days (or more) per week. If needed, you can break the exercise into multiple ten- to fifteen-minute segments. Find activities that you enjoy—whether it is walking, a Zumba class, swimming, or bicycling. In fact, you may want to vary your routine to keep it interesting. If you are overly fatigued, consider laying off for a day, but be careful not to break your routine for long.

As you begin your program, be aware of how you feel and whether there is a need to make modifications. You want to find forms of exercise that actively engage you, making the time spent more a joy and less a drudgery.

EXTENDING EXERCISE BEYOND THE TREATMENT HORIZON

Exercise may be as important to the cancer survivor as it is during active treatment, so just because you have finished treatment or are in remission, don't abandon the gym!

SUPPLEMENTAL READING

We are asking you to make a substantial and ongoing investment of time and energy in exercise. Like any investment, you may wish to do some additional research before proceeding. There are many excellent books detailing the health benefits of exercise. Here are a few for your consideration:

- *Spark: The Revolutionary New Science of Exercise and the Brain*, by John J. Ratey
- *ACSM's Guide to Exercise and Cancer Survivorship*, edited by Melinda L. Irwin
- *The Breast Cancer Survivor's Fitness Plan: A Doctor-Approved Workout Plan for a Strong Body and Lifesaving Results* (Harvard Medical School Guides), by Carolyn M. Kaelin, Francesca Coltrera, Josie Gardiner, and Joy Prouty
- *What Makes Olga Run? The Mystery of the 90-Something Track Star and What She Can Teach Us about Living Longer, Happier Lives*, by Bruce Grierson

- *Lifelong Running: Overcome the 11 Myths about Running and Live a Healthier Life*, by Ruth Heidrich
- *Exercise for Mood and Anxiety: Proven Strategies for Overcoming Depression and Enhancing Well-Being*, by Michael W. Otto and Jasper A. J. Smits

YOUR GOALS

Remember: Through a little effort, there is much to be gained, including:

- improved physical health;
- reduced impact of certain side effects;
- greater strength, flexibility, and balance—depending on the types of exercise you choose to engage in;
- improved well-being and a direct reduction in your level of distress;
- improved tolerance for treatments; and
- the potential for an improved prognosis.

I hope we have provided you with sufficient encouragement to consider exercising regularly. It can make a significant difference in the quality of your life and potentially even your outcome.

11

WHAT TO EXPECT FROM PAIN CONTROL

Physicians often refer to pain as the fifth vital sign—an acknowledgement of its significance to your health and well-being. Pain can dramatically affect a patient's quality of life. Furthermore, uncontrolled pain is among cancer patients' greatest fears.

While there is no denying that the pain from certain types of cancer can be intense, physicians have the ability to manage it in most cases. For such management to occur, it is essential that patients have some understanding of pain and that there is excellent communication between the patient, caregiver, and physician regarding their pain.

DEFINING *PAIN*

While all of us know pain when we experience it, it's helpful to have an agreed-upon definition. Here is one that Lori and I find helpful:

> Pain is a sensation of discomfort, distress, or agony. It may be acute or chronic. Acute pain is moderate to severe and lasts a relatively short time (usually less than three months). It is usually a signal that body tissue is being injured in some way, and it generally disappears when the injury heals. Chronic pain may range from mild to severe, and is present to some degree for longer periods of time (generally lasting longer than three to six months). Because pain is unique to each individual, a person's pain cannot be evaluated by someone else. [1]

DESCRIBING PAIN

Your physician's ability to help manage your pain is enhanced by your ability to describe it precisely. Such words such as *dull, throbbing, sharp, burning,* and *steady,* when accompanied by information about *frequency, duration,* and *intensity,* provide important information that your physician can translate into a pain management plan. In an effort to standardize how pain is described, the National Cancer Institute (NCI) suggests using a short list of words, including:

- dull pain—a slow or weak pain, not very sudden or strong.
- throbbing pain—a pain that surges, beats, or pounds.
- steady pain—a pain that does not change in its intensity.
- sharp pain—pain that causes intense mental or physical distress.
- acute pain—severe pain that lasts a relatively short period of time.
- chronic or persistent pain—mild to severe pain that is present to some degree for long periods of time.
- breakthrough pain—when you are taking medication for chronic pain, moderate to severe pain that occurs between doses (pain that "breaks through").[2]

In addition to these descriptive terms, your physician may have questions that help him or her determine the best ways to address your pain, for example:

- When did you first experience pain?
- What is the duration of the pain?
- Where precisely is the pain located?
- How intense is the pain?
- Has the nature of the pain changed?
- What makes the pain better or worse?
- Is the pain worse during certain times of the day or night?[3]

The more accurately you report your symptoms, the better your physician is able to do his or her job. Hence, patients are advised to keep notes or a journal that provide a concise synopsis of their symptoms, including whether their pain responded to medication. The NCI specifically advises patients:

Write down the details of any discomfort you might have been having so you will not forget to report them. Consider keeping a diary of your pain, or ask a friend or family member to help track your symptoms. The types of information that you may want to note in your diary include:

- date
- time
- pain scale rating
- type and dose of medication
- time pain medication was taken
- how well pain responded to medication taken
- any other pain relief methods attempted

Your physician may need to refer to your diary when making a plan to relieve your pain and to make you more comfortable, therefore, be sure to bring it with you to your physician visits.[4]

Lori has found several other factors to be important in understanding and managing a patient's pain, including:

- conditions that exacerbate or relieve the pain and
- whether the pain is focused in one or two locations or travels to different sites within the body.

MEASURING AND ASSESSING PAIN

Your doctor may ask about any pain you are experiencing at the time of your initial visit, as well as throughout the treatment process. Health care professionals employ a simple method of evaluating the severity of pain using a scale calibrated from 1 to 10. Patients are shown a scale, which generally features illustrations of faces showing relative levels of distress, and are asked to assign a number to their pain. A rating of 1 would correspond with minimal pain barely worthy of note, whereas a rating of 10 would indicate the worst pain you have ever experienced or unbearable pain. Lori adds that a patient's pain could be so intense that, when first asked to describe it, they respond, "It's an 11," or "It's a 15." In other words, it's off the chart. These patients need immediate attention. She stresses that it will aid your physician tremendously if you provide an accurate description of your pain.

As part of your pain assessment, your doctor may elect to check you for any physical indicators of problems contributing to your pain as well as review your health and medical history. In addition, he or she may perform a neurological examination that includes a "series of questions and tests to check the brain, spinal cord, and nerve function. The exam checks your mental status, coordination, and ability to walk normally, and how well the muscles, senses, and reflexes work."[5]

WHAT CAUSES THE PAIN THAT OFTEN ACCOMPANIES CANCER?

There can be numerous underlying causes of pain. Sometimes the cause is readily apparent, whereas other times the pain is more idiopathic in nature—without an identifiable source. If the pain is persistent, it is important that you speak with your physician.

Potential causes of unremitting cancer pain include:

- growth of a tumor, resulting in pressure on various parts of the body, including organs, bones, and nerves;
- metastatic spread of the cancer within the body;
- impaired circulation;
- blockages within the body, including such areas as colon, bile duct, bladder, and other organs;
- infection, including sepsis;
- swelling;
- side effects of treatment; and
- psychological distress[6]

It is important to note that psychological stress can cause pain or exacerbate pain brought on by physical conditions—all the more reason distress needs to be actively managed in cancer patients in addition to pain.

TYPES OF PAIN

Patients who have cancerous tumors within their bones experience a different sensation of pain than patients who have a tumor impinging on major nerves or the spinal cord. It is important to recognize that these different types of pain are responsive to selective interventions.

WHAT TREATMENTS ARE AVAILABLE?

Physicians' first line of defense against pain is most often medications. For minor to moderate pain, over-the-counter medications can prove helpful. Although they are not without both risks and side effects, such drugs as ibuprofen, aspirin, and acetaminophen are generally safer than more potent pain relievers.

As pain escalates on the scale of 1 to 10, so, too, will the intensity of the medicine your physician prescribes. The most frequently prescribed class of drugs for managing moderate to severe pain are opioids (derived from opium). Opioids range exponentially in strength from moderately analgesic compounds, such as hydrocodone, to extremely potent drugs like fentanyl.

Each drug has a very precise dose as well as frequency with which the medication may be taken. Some drugs are designed to be fast acting but relatively short lived in terms of duration, whereas others provide sustained pain relief over time (long acting). The method by which the drug is administered (such as oral or a time-released patch) also impacts the frequency with which it must be taken.

Certain antidepressants also have the capacity to inhibit pain. Both SSRIs (selective serotonin reuptake inhibitors) and SNRIs (selective norepinephrine reuptake inhibitors) appear to help modulate pain in many patients when there is a neural component to the pain. The drugs can be given exclusively or in conjunction with other medications.

Your physicians may also suggest a palliative consult or a pain management consult. Palliative physicians specialize in managing the pain that accompanies a number of disease processes. Some patients mistakenly assume that seeing a palliative specialist means that the end must be near. While palliative specialists are quite versed in hospice care, they are also very skilled in working with patients over extended periods of time to manage their pain. Pain management physicians are usually anesthesiologists who subspecialize in managing acute and chronic pain through interventions and medications. If your physician recommends a pain specialist or a palliative consult, you have nothing to lose and probably much to gain by complying.

COMMON SIDE EFFECTS OF MEDICATIONS

All medications carry the risk of side effects. Ibuprofen can impair kidney function, aspirin carries the risk of stomach bleeding, and acetaminophen can be toxic to the liver—particularly when combined with alcohol or taken consistently over extended periods of time.

The opioids are sedating in certain doses, constipating, and can cause nausea. Often these side effects either diminish in intensity or abate after taking the medication for a short time. Opioids also carry the potential for abuse, addiction, and overdose, although such problems are extremely infrequent in cancer patients. Unfortunately, opioid abuse in the general population has resulted in efforts to curtail the usage of many of these drugs—drugs that can prove invaluable to cancer patients.

The antidepressants carry an array of risks ranging from increased suicidal thinking to problems with sexual potency. Certain drugs can also carry metabolic risks, such as increasing your propensity to develop diabetes.

It should be very clear that powerful medications can, indeed, alleviate suffering, but they can also induce it. As such, they must be used with great care under the oversight of your physicians.

TOO MANY COOKS IN THE KITCHEN

If you are like most cancer patients, you have a team of doctors who are responsible for your treatment. While generally quite beneficial to the patient, this departmentalization of care can result in patients receiving duplicative or synergistic interventions and medications for their pain. Not only is this an ineffective way of managing pain, but also the lack of coordination puts the patient at risk for potentially serious side effects.

Lori has made it a practice to ensure that one physician on the team assumes responsibility for the important task of managing a patient's pain. She also counsels that the patient should take responsibility for maintaining an accurate and up-to-date list of over-the-counter and prescription medications and ensuring that all physicians have a current copy of it.

METHODS OF DRUG DELIVERY: ADVANTAGES AND DISADVANTAGES

Different medications prescribed to manage your pain may require different methods of administration. Most over-the-counter medications are orally administered, as are many prescription pain relievers.

Some medications, however, require alternative methods of delivery. When rapid relief is required, you may receive an injection. Injections may be under the skin, known as *subcutaneous*, directly into a vein (*intravenous*), or into the fluid-filled cavity surrounding the spinal cord, as is the case with "intraspinal opioids [that] are injected into the fluid around the spinal cord. These may be combined with a local anesthetic to help some patients who have pain that is very hard to control."[7]

When sustained pain management is required over extended periods of time, your physician may prescribe patches. When applied to the skin, these patches allow the continual administration of a medication over hours or days. The patches can be combined with oral or other forms of medication as needed.

Patients who are unable to swallow pills or capsules may be prescribed suppositories or skin creams. Many of the more common analgesics are available in this form.

If pain is severe enough to warrant a constant infusion of medication into the bloodstream, a pain pump may be inserted into the patient's IV line.

Patient-controlled analgesia (PCA) pumps are one way to control pain through your IV line. A PCA pump allows the patient to control the amount of drug that is used. With a PCA pump, you can receive a preset opioid dose by pressing a button on a computerized pump that is connected to a small tube. Once the pain is controlled, the doctor may prescribe regular opioid doses based on the amount you used with the PCA pump.[8]

RADIATION TO AMELIORATE PAIN

Radiation can be used to ameliorate (or *palliate*) pain. It can be particularly effective in mitigating bone pain created by metastases (cancer cells that have spread from the primary tumor to a distant site) to the bone. Another important use of radiation is to treat tumors impinging on the spinal cord. This condition can not only cause grievous pain but also paralysis if left untreated. Radiation helps rapidly shrink the tumor and reduce its pressure on the spinal cord.

Various types of radiation are used to palliate pain. Most forms of palliative radiation involve the use of an external beam focused precisely on the sources of pain. Depending on the type of equipment used, these treatments may require a few or numerous treatments over days and weeks.

Another form of palliative radiation therapy takes the form of an injection of radioactive isotopes. The specific isotopes are selected based on the manner in which they are absorbed by the human body. Once absorbed, the radiative isotope emits energy that can destroy cancer cells lodged deep within bone.

OTHER WAYS TO CONTROL PAIN

Your physician is not limited to medicines and radiation to help control your pain. Other potent methods of pain control include:

- **Radio-Frequency Ablation (RFA).** RFA can create tremendous heat that selectively destroys tissue without the need to operate. As such, it can be used to target structures that are contributing to significant pain.
- **Neurological Treatments.** "Surgery can be done to implant a device that delivers drugs or stimulates the nerves with mild electric current. In rare cases, surgery may be done to destroy a nerve or nerves that are part of the pain pathway."[9]

- **Nerve Blocks.** "A nerve block is the injection of either a local anesthetic or a drug into or around a nerve to block pain. Nerve blocks help control pain that can't be controlled in other ways. Nerve blocks may also be used to find where the pain is coming from, to predict how the pain will respond to long-term treatments, and to prevent pain after certain procedures."[10]

Highly trained surgical, radiology, and anesthesiology specialists deliver these types of interventions. Your oncologist will be able to help direct you to the right specialist for your condition.

LESS INVASIVE METHODS OF MANAGING PAIN

Exercise can be a potent form of pain relief for some patients while also reducing anxiety and depression that exacerbate pain. It is important to have a prescribed exercise plan that has been approved by your physician before embarking on a new program, as described in chapter 10.

Some patients have found that various complementary therapies are effective in addressing their pain. Acupuncture works well for some patients. Others find that the relaxation resulting from therapeutic massage or yoga brings a level of relief. Talk to your physician before engaging in complementary modalities to ensure that he or she has no concerns with such actions. Most physicians will be supportive if the complementary modality does not put you at additional risk.

Many of the standard treatments used for athletic injuries can also bring a modicum of pain relief. For instance, both heat and cold can be therapeutic in reducing pain and inflammation.

Some patients are further aided by various types of psychosocial support that help them relax or receive empathic responses to their situations.

TO LEARN MORE ABOUT PAIN MANAGEMENT

Pain management is an essential topic for most cancer patients, and we have provided you with only the briefest of overviews. You may wish to do some supplemental reading on the topic. A good book to begin with is *A Nation in Pain: Healing Our Biggest Health Problem.*[11]

12

HOW TO MANAGE THE COST OF CANCER

Cancer takes more than a physical toll. It also takes a financial toll. More than $86 billion was spent on cancer care in America in 2009. Studies predict that this number will soar to $157 billion by 2020.[1] If drug companies continue to raise the prices of cancer therapeutics, the number will grow even larger. When you add in the additional indirect costs associated with cancer, the costs more than double.[2]

These are not pie-in-the-sky numbers but rather costs that affect every cancer patient and his or her family in America. These costs wreak financial havoc on many families, even leading to bankruptcy. In fact, health care costs have been one of the leading causes of bankruptcy in America for a number of years.[3]

The goal, therefore, is not only to survive the physical ravages of cancer but also to manage the costs of your treatment to the best of your ability.

UNDERSTANDING THE COST OF TREATMENT

It is essential that you understand the cost of your proposed treatment. A first step is to meet with financial counselors to understand your obligations based on the projected cost of your treatment. Because the journey through cancer is unpredictable, no one can tell you precisely what treatment will cost. However, a financial counselor who is aligned with the facility at which you will be receiving care should be able to define:

- projected costs for your initial treatment(s);
- costs for prescribed chemotherapeutic agents, as well as pre-scribed medications;
- anticipated costs for follow-up scans or tests; and
- other costs frequently incurred in cases such as yours.

Just as importantly, the financial counselor should have the requisite skills to decode your insurance coverage, helping you to understand clearly what types of expenses are covered, to what extent, and how this translates into out-of-pocket expenses for you.

I had the pleasure of meeting with Julia S., a financial counselor at a major university-affiliated cancer center. According to Julia, "Most people are not expecting the high out-of-pocket expenses they are going to incur. They are not prepared financially for the high cost of cancer. Surprisingly, many people do not know what they have for benefits. I would strongly suggest that people understand their benefits and what might be needed for adequate coverage."[4]

Insurance is confusing enough without being overwhelmed by a diagnosis of cancer. Julia indicated that some patients struggle to take in what she is sharing with them: "Some people seem to take it really well; they know what their benefits are before I tell them. And then some people are overwhelmed with everything else they are dealing with." That is why she recommends that patients "have someone else with them to help gather information. I think it is important for the patient to bring someone with them to these meetings. More than 85 percent do."[5]

Rhonda C., a medical social worker who shares patients with Julia, is in full agreement with the importance of having family members or other caregivers present when discussing how to meet the financial challenges of cancer: "Having a support person is extremely important in determining how well they will do with their cancer treatment in total."[6]

WHAT IS MY DOCTOR'S ROLE IN MANAGING THE COST OF MY TREATMENT?

Remember that your doctor is trained to treat your cancer, not manage the financial ramifications of that treatment. Dr. S. Yousuf Zafar, a physician at the Duke Cancer Institute, summed it up this way in a powerful post in the *ASCO Connection* newsletter:

> As oncologists, we painstakingly translate clinical evidence for our patients. We inform them of odds, percentages, risks, and survival. When it comes to deciding on a treatment path, we lean heavily on the potential of physical toxicity, as we should, but are we missing the elephant in the room? Cancer treatment is among the most expensive forms of treatment, costing over $200 billion per year in just the United States. In this era of cost-sharing, when patients are taking on a greater burden of health care costs, we have to wonder how that mind-boggling number filters down into the daily lives of our patients. The evidence suggests that even patients with insurance are struggling to make ends meet; national estimates of out-of-pocket expenditures for patients with cancer fall in the range of $4,000 to $5,000 per year. In order to defray medical expenses, patients with cancer are spending their savings, cutting back on food and clothing, and being non-adherent to medications, including chemotherapy.[7]

Dr. Zafar reminds his readers that most doctors are uncomfortable discussing financial matters with their patients. Also, he goes on to provide excellent, three-point guidance to physicians—advice that may be helpful to you, the patient:

> First, we have to address cost even with less-than-sufficient data for a truly informed discussion. Without price transparency, we cannot hope to provide patients with complete cost information. However, lack of price transparency should not prevent us altogether from helping our patients with their financial burden. Asking a pharmacist to assess patients' insurance coverage before they fill expensive prescriptions is useful. While I might not be able to tell a patient exactly how much their oral chemotherapy will cost, I can turn to team members who can access that data.
>
> Second, we must provide patients with the opportunity to consider alternatives and make trade-offs. Most patients realize that they will incur some costs as a result of their cancer treatment, and most

patients are willing to bear some financial burden. However, not all patients have the same priorities. We must start thinking critically and creatively about the value in the treatments we provide. Compared to forging ahead with the next line of therapy, we may find it more difficult to inform a patient about the alternative of not receiving chemotherapy. But we might be doing them a much greater service in allowing them to consider a trade-off. Less challenging means to cost reduction include less frequent imaging, fewer tests, and less expensive supportive care drugs. . . .

Finally, the sensitive nature of finances is often a barrier to cost discussions between patients and doctors. This combined with our less-than-complete education around how to talk costs can make for an uncomfortable conversation. In the outcome-oriented, data driven world of oncology, talking about costs without a solution in mind can seem counterintuitive. However, just acknowledging the patient's struggle with costs can provide some relief in knowing that their doctors are aware of their situation. We can find an analogy in discussions about end-of-life care. While we cannot often "fix" what patients and their families experience near the end of life, we can validate their concerns and help where we can. As this topic comes up more frequently, oncologists should be aware of helpful resources, including pharmaceutical funds, foundation support, and nonprofit organizations such as the American Cancer Society and Cancer Support Community. ASCO provides information for patients on managing the cost of cancer care at Cancer.Net. These organizations have collected resources for patients with specific financial needs (e.g., copayment assistance, travel assistance), and patients are often unaware of these resources.[8]

Rhonda C. says that physicians often misinterpret a patient's apprehension over cost as resistance or noncompliance with the doctor's recommendation: "What may look like resistance to the doctor [relative to a treatment recommendation] may really be fear on the part of the patient about the costs of treatment."[9] What is needed is good, straightforward communication between parties.

FEAR ABOUT THE ABILITY TO AFFORD NEEDED CARE

It is quite understandable that among cancer patients' greatest fears are how they will afford their treatment and the impact that the costs associated with their disease will have on them and their families. A survey conducted in 2009 by the Association of Oncology Social Work clearly demonstrated that patients' fears had a profound impact on their lives:

> According to the survey, 66% of patients with major financial challenges suffer depression or anxiety, 29% delay filling prescriptions due to financial pressures, and 22% skip doses of their medications. Sixty-three percent of oncology social workers surveyed said financial issues reduce patients' compliance with their cancer treatment even though that treatment is key to their recovery. Additionally, 40% of patients reported depleting their savings, almost 30% reported dealing with bill collectors, and 54% of those handling a major/catastrophic financial burden said it had become more difficult in the past year to afford treatment.
>
> Furthermore, 68% of cancer patients and caregivers surveyed reported that the patient is experiencing financial hardship due to medical bills, and 55% of all cancer patients surveyed said the stress of dealing with costs negatively affects their ability to focus on their recovery.[10]

The fear is justifiable, and the best way to manage it, as Julia shared, is by being fully informed and understanding what is within one's realm to control.

In addition to speaking with a financial counselor, Julia advises that patients meet with a social worker: "A social worker can help with applications for social security disability or housing assistance, transportation, or prescription assistance. There are a lot of programs within hospital systems that patients may not be aware of."[11]

WHAT WILL MY INSURANCE COVER?

It is important that you understand precisely what your insurance will cover. Often patients find out too late that their insurance either limits their ability to seek care from their provider of choice or provides an insufficient benefit to make treatment affordable.

MANAGING YOUR MANAGED CARE ORGANIZATION (MCO)

If you thought dealing with cancer was difficult, just wait until you have to deal with your insurance or MCO. We say this only somewhat face-tiously. Here's a quick insight gleaned from a research study examining problems encountered by breast cancer patients when interacting with their MCOs:

> Interviews of patients with breast cancer revealed that interactions with managed care organizations (MCOs), including issues with bill-ing accuracy, copayments, and referrals, were a major burden and affected perceptions of the quality of care. Two major themes emerged from this research. The first was that patients had "difficul-ty completing managed care tasks" (involving issues such as getting a referral; clarifying copayment levels; finding knowledgeable and helpful MCO staff; and getting assistance with paperwork, billing, and treatment approvals). In addition, patients perceived a lack of logical and caring decision making on the part of the MCO. Delays in determining out-of-pocket expenses resulted in distress and difficul-ty in planning future treatments.
>
> In addition to the physical vulnerability associated with their con-dition, patients were subject to a financial vulnerability related to payment for care, because they worried about discontinuation of coverage and inability to get further treatment if coverage was dis-continued. Most patients expressed a lack of confidence that there would be improvements in the MCO system over time.
>
> The second major theme was problems in "managing or mediat-ing between the MCO and the cancer [care providers]," in which patients perceived MCO management and cancer care as separate entities that had to be linked by the patient to achieve the best outcomes. Whereas some patients accepted assistance from the can-cer center about billing issues when possible, others used a more take-charge approach and expressed frustration at the extra level of complication caused by this paperwork. In addition, patients felt bur-dened with having to coordinate between the provider and the payer while also taking care of their physical needs related to the disease.
>
> A study by Bourjolly and colleagues that involved interviews with 33 women who had breast cancer revealed main areas of difficulty with insurance: obtaining referrals and receiving medical services in different locations. The patients' primary concern was finding the

best care to treat their disease regardless of the type of insurance they had. Having to get referrals was regarded as a very frustrating experience.[12]

Lori and I recommend that you take advantage of a financial counselor's willingness to run interference with your insurance company/MCO. Also seek out a social worker, if one is available through your provider, who can identify sources of financial assistance for noninsurance-related needs. These counselors are experienced experts who can deftly manage the difficult job of ensuring your benefits are properly realized.

WHEN YOUR INSURANCE COMPANY REFUSES TO COVER A PROPOSED TREATMENT

Your insurance company may refuse to provide coverage because a proposed treatment is not deemed medically indicated or necessary. In essence, they are questioning your physician's judgment, which may or may not be warranted. Either way, it is disruptive to care. When this happens, Julia S. told me, "There are three options: (1) Patients can talk to their doctor about an alternative treatment; (2) they can appeal the decision; (3) they can elect to go forward with the knowledge that their treatment will not be covered, in which case the patient will be fully liable for the cost."[13]

Sometimes a treatment is denied after it is completed. In this case, Julia said, "If it is denied after the fact, we will write off the charges. That is our contractual obligation with the insurance company."[14]

TIMES ARE CHANGING

Lori has observed changes over the past several years in the frequency with which insurance companies deny approval for tests or treatments recommended by physicians. Though there is an appeals process for such denials, it can be extremely cumbersome and frustrating. At the very least, it often delays care. Lori adds, "As a physician, I find it difficult to find the time to appeal an insurance denial. They are hoping you will just give up. However, I will always go to bat for my patients when I feel that it is the right thing to do, as will most of my colleagues."

OTHER FORMS OF FINANCIAL ASSISTANCE

There may be other forms of financial assistance available for patients in addition to insurance. Such assistance usually takes one of three forms: (1) grants available within the community to help defray out-of-pocket costs for cancer patients, (2) hospital/clinical/health system programs or policies to help patients in financial need, and (3) programs sponsored by pharmaceutical firms to make their drugs more affordable to patients meeting certain criteria.

A financial counselor or social worker can help you identify the forms of assistance you may qualify to receive. The criteria can include not only your financial status but also whether you are covered by private insurance or such governmental programs as Medicare or have no insurance coverage.

As an experienced financial counselor, Rhonda C. has become quite creative in cobbling together various forms of financial assistance to aid patients in need. When I asked Rhonda what advice she would give to patients being treated at facilities that do not offer social workers or financial counselors, she suggested:

> Start by seeing if your county has a cancer coalition or some way to link to community support for cancer patients. Most communities have such services now. These coalitions generally help with medication assistance, transportation assistance, even reimbursement for gas required to visit the doctor. They usually have emotional support available, including either social workers on staff or linkages to social workers in the community.[15]

Do not be prideful or shy about asking for assistance. Costs continue to skyrocket, and you should take advantage of any opportunity to lower your direct costs of treatment.

NEWER FORMS OF THERAPY DRIVE UP THE COSTS

Thanks to tremendous scientific advancements in the fields of genomics, proteomics, and molecular biology, commonly referred to as *personalized medicine*, researchers have developed a host of new diagnostic and chemotherapeutic treatments capable of more precisely targeting and controlling certain types of cancer. Some of these chemotherapeutic agents have proven to be nothing short of miraculous. One of the best examples is Gleevec, a drug first approved in 2001 for the treatment of chronic myelogenous leukemia and now approved for use with certain types of solid tumors: "Gleevec entered the market in 2001 at a price of about $30,000 a year in the United States. . . . Since then, the price has tripled . . . even as Gleevec has faced competition from five newer drugs. And those drugs are even more expensive."[16] It does not take a tremendous volume of patients to hit a home run in drug sales. In 2012, Gleevec became the top-selling drug at Novartis, racking up $4.7 billion in sales.[17]

PROFITING ON THE BACKS OF CANCER PATIENTS

Please forgive me while I stand briefly on my soapbox. I feel compelled to make you aware of certain practices by the pharmaceutical industry that Lori and I believe to be highly unethical. While such drugs as Gleevec (imatinib) can literally be lifesavers, they come at a dear price. Pharmaceutical companies are quick to recognize the profit potential inherent in these drugs and price them accordingly: "Imatinib was developed as a 'goodwill gesture' by Novartis, and became a blockbuster, with annual revenues of about $4.7 billion in 2012. As one of the most successful cancer targeted therapies, imatinib may have set the pace for the rising cost of cancer drugs."[18]

A report published in May 2014 by the IMS Institute for Healthcare Informatics stated, "The average cost per month of branded oncology drug treatment in the U.S. is now about $10,000, up from an average of $5,000 a decade ago."[19] Based on this finding, it is easy to see how eleven of the twelve drugs approved by the FDA for cancer treatment in 2012 cost more than $100,000 per year per patient.[20] The cost of drugs has become a highly contentious issue, particularly in the United

States, where we consume 41 percent of all oncology drug sales world-wide. [21]

Pharmaceutical manufacturers are clearly betting on oncology drugs for a strong return to their bottom line: "Cancer remains the biggest portion of the overall drug development pipeline in earlier phases with four times the number of drugs in the pipeline than the next therapeutic class." [22] While we are praying for drug breakthroughs that bring new hope to cancer patients, drug company executives are hoping for higher quarterly earnings that help to raise their stock prices.

Fortunately, there are growing efforts to keep escalating prices in check. An increasing number of leading oncologists are challenging the major pharmaceutical firms to set fair prices for their products: "As physicians, we follow the Hippocratic Oath of 'Primum non nocere,' first (or above all) do no harm. We believe the unsustainable drug prices in CML and cancer may be causing harm to patients. Advocating for lower drug prices is a necessity to save the lives of patients who cannot afford them." [23]

Major physician organizations, such as the American Society for Clinical Oncology (ASCO), are working to develop mechanisms for analyzing the relative value of new drugs by examining such factors as improvements in efficacy, reduction of side effects, ease of administration, and so forth. These guidelines will then help medical oncologists make value-based recommendations to their patients.

Finally, insurance companies are actively exploring ways to reduce cost. The Brookings Institute, in an article published in June 2014, provided these examples:

> Several health plans and providers are already showing results. A Pennsylvania-based collaboration with the University of Pittsburgh Medical Center and commercial payers achieved savings of more than $1 million in only six months by controlling and reducing the use of Avastin through clinical pathways. A Washington-based health plan also achieved $1 million in cost savings through a partnership with 22 medical oncologists. Most recently, one of the nation's largest health plans announced a new clinical pathways program that provides oncologists with $350 per patient per month (PMPM) for adhering to specific chemotherapy regimens. The program will be rolled out in July across six states with potential for expansion after its first year. [24]

Only time will tell how pharmaceutical executives will respond to this call for fair pricing. In the interim, many patients will struggle to find ways of paying for needed medications.

CHECKING THE PRICE FOR OTHER PRESCRIPTION DRUGS USED WITH CANCER TREATMENT

Many different types of drugs are used in cancer treatment in addition to the cancer-specific agent. There are drugs to prevent nausea, treat pain, help with anxiety, or control diarrhea. Drug prices can vary a lot. You (or a family member) may want to call different pharmacies in an effort to find the best price.

When your doctor prescribes medicines or outpatient care, here are some questions you may want to ask:

- If I get outpatient treatment, how much of it will be covered by my health insurance?
- How much will the chemotherapy drug that I take by mouth cost me? What about the nausea medicines and other drugs that go along with it? How much will I have to pay for this drug? Will my insurance cover it? (Ask this about each prescription given.)
- Are there assistance programs to help me get the drugs I need?
- Are there less expensive drugs or generic forms that work as well?
- Is there any other way I can get help paying for this drug?[25]

WHEN TRADE-OFFS BETWEEN "OPTIMAL" CARE AND AFFORDABILITY ARE NECESSARY

Your physician needs to understand the financial constraints governing your treatment. He or she may be able to offer appropriate alternatives to the highly expensive treatments. Your physician will also be able to explain what the potential trade-offs are in terms of treatment effectiveness, immediate and longer-term side effects, and convenience.

Here is what Lori has to say on this matter:

> If I recommend radiation therapy to a patient with a high copay or other out-of-pocket expense, I try to work with them to reduce that

burden if they are stressed about cost. For instance, the number of treatments and the way they are timed may make a huge difference in the patient's out-of-pocket expense. We can work on timing to make treatment more affordable.

If my patient is not able to afford a specific medication, I would rather prescribe one they can afford even if it is not my number one choice. Taking needed medication is always better than no medication.

As a patient, please inform your physician if you have financial concerns. Chances are he or she will be more than happy to work with you on a solution.

BILLING CHALLENGES

Medical bills appear to be written in the most impenetrable code imaginable. Mere mortals find it almost impossible to decipher charges associated with their cancer treatments. Thus, they have difficulty even verifying that the charges are correct, which is problematic because bills are often in error.

Here, Julia offers some straightforward advice: "You need to look at your explanation of benefits, which most insurance companies will provide. If you compare this with your bill, it should match up. If it does not, there may be an error either on the part of the provider or the insurance company. Always check your explanation of benefits against your bill!"[26]

QUESTIONS TO ASK

The American Cancer Society's website provides a list of important questions to ask your various providers of care, including:

- Do we need to get my insurance company's approval (sometimes called pre-certification) before the test, surgery, treatment, home care, etc.?
- Is there a co-pay for each treatment session? (The co-pay is a cost you will be charged each time you get chemo, radiation, intrave-

nous [IV] antibiotics, IV fluids, or other outpatient treatments that you get in an office or clinic. The co-pay amount is set by your health insurance company.)

- If I must go into the hospital, how much will it cost? How much will my insurance cover?
- Is there a way to know beforehand if the doctors who will see me in the hospital are in my health plan network?
- Counting all the charges (hospital, anesthesia, surgeon, pathologist, and more), how much will this surgery cost me? How much will my insurance cover?
- Should I plan for rehab, home care, or long-term care (such as nursing home or hospice care)?[27]

SAYING THE SERENITY PRAYER

Many of the financial implications of cancer are simply beyond your control. While it is essential that you do your best to understand the costs you are likely to incur and the degree to which these costs will be offset by insurance, it is equally important that you push to get the care you need and deserve. Recognize what is and is not within your ability to control, and let go of ruminating over things that you cannot change.

13

WHEN CONSIDERING COMPLEMENTARY THERAPIES

Mary E., like many cancer patients, included complementary medicine as part of her journey through cancer. She was not seeking a novel way to eliminate the disease but rather exploring ways to improve her quality of life: "Prior to my surgery, I had Reiki. Whether it helped or not, I can't say. To me, there's not just the physical body, but a spirit also. I think the spirit needs encouragement and help along the way, too. I also did a facial, just to make me feel relaxed during treatment."[1]

WHAT IS MEANT BY "COMPLEMENTARY" THERAPIES?

Because complementary therapies often play a role in a cancer patient's treatment regimen, it is important that they be well understood, beginning with their definition:

> CAM [complementary and alternative medicine] is defined by the National Center for Complementary and Alternative Medicine as "a group of diverse medical and health care systems, practices, and products that are not presently considered to be part of conventional medicine," a definition that remains fluid as more complementary therapies become incorporated into conventional care (e.g., massage and acupuncture).[2]

The five most utilized forms of CAM by cancer patients include:

1. vitamin/mineral supplements (76.64 percent),
2. prayer for self (68.85 percent),
3. intercessory prayer (49.22%),
4. chiropractic/osteopathic manipulation (34.60%), and
5. herbal therapies (32.14%).[3]

COMPLEMENTARY VERSUS ALTERNATIVE

Complementary therapies do not replace or supplant traditional methods of managing cancer. Rather, they are intended to provide additional benefits to the cancer patient, which can vary from reducing the adverse side effects of treatment to attempting to bolster the patient's immune response. They are thus intended to complement standard oncology practices.

The term *alternative therapies* suggests that these interventions are done in lieu of medical treatment—an obviously risky decision, particularly if there are effective treatment modalities available for your cancer. Yet, even some of the brightest people on the planet have chosen to forgo standard medical therapy in pursuit of alternative treatment:

> Giving up conventional medicine in favour of alternative treatments, tops the list of fatefully wrong decisions. Whenever this has hastened the death of a famous individual, like recently Steve Jobs, the world press briefly takes notice only to revert to "business as usual" a few days later. And "business as usual" means all too often the promotion of quackery to desperate patients. Thankfully, most cancer patients do not abandon conventional oncology but use alternative treatments as an adjunct to it.[4]

One of the preeminent experts on complementary medicine, Barrie Cassileth, is crystal clear in her opinion regarding the role of alternative medicine in cancer care—there is none! Dr. Cassileth, who is the founder of Memorial Sloan-Kettering's integrative medicine program, offered these thoughts in an interview with Medscape journalist Gabriel Miller:

> The most common misconception and misperception is that there is a relationship between alternative therapies and complementary

therapies, which are part of integrative medicine. There are no viable alternatives to mainstream cancer care, but there are many products and services that are sold to the public, to the naive public, calling themselves alternative medicines or alternative therapies. . . . All of this is bogus. There are no viable alternatives to mainstream care, but a lot of people are getting wealthy pushing alternatives. In other words, they say, "Don't bother with mainstream treatment; you don't have to get surgery or chemotherapy or whatever. Come here, and we will treat you." With something that turns out to be utter nonsense. What happens to these patients. . . . They usually die because they failed to get treatment when it was needed. That is alternative medicine. No one who is a reliable person at a reliable institution would have anything to do with alternative medicine, also called quackery.[5]

Most physicians would agree with Dr. Cassileth, so don't expect your doctor to turn cartwheels if you elect to forgo traditional medical care in favor of alternative medicine. It should be noted that, despite the significant difference between complementary and alternative medicine, they are often spoken of together as differing from traditional or allopathic medicine.

WHY DO PATIENTS SEEK OUT THIS TYPE OF CARE?

There are numerous reasons that some patients seek out complementary and alternative medicine. Some patients are simply seeking ways to improve their quality of life during treatment; others are searching for an elusive cure. Still others are "motivated to try various complementary and alternative modalities by well-wishing family members, friends, other cancer patients and survivors."[6]

Patients undergoing active treatment, as well as survivors post-treatment, use CAM therapies. Cancer survivors seek out CAM for many of the same reasons as patients undergoing active treatment:

Many cancer survivors turn to CAM therapies in addition to their conventional treatment to deal with health issues such as recurring pain, insomnia, and ongoing psychological distress. Cancer survivors report that they seek CAM in order to gain a sense of control, to manage symptoms, to improve quality of life, and to boost the immune system. Cancer survivors may also seek CAM because they desire non-pharmacologic therapies to treat their symptoms or deal with needs that are unmet by conventional medical care.[7]

It is difficult to ascertain precisely how many cancer patients are using CAM due to the ambiguity of the term *CAM*. When it includes such things as prayer, meditation, and the use of supplements, the number of users increases dramatically—perhaps more than doubling. Here are the findings from one major study:

> A total of 1,755 surveys were available for analysis, of which 1,228 (71.5%) respondents indicated a cancer diagnosis. Among those with a cancer diagnosis, 75.2% (n = 923) were currently using at least one CAM modality, and 57.6% (n = 532) of CAM users initiated use after diagnosis. Of those who initiated CAM after cancer diagnosis, 93.2% (n = 496) were still using CAM at the time of the survey.[8]

WHO USES CAM MOST FREQUENTLY?

Research has also helped identify those patients most likely to use CAM therapies: "Predictors of higher CAM use by patients with cancer include female gender, stage of disease at diagnosis, age, higher education, higher income, race, and geographical location. Additionally, individuals living at a greater distance from health care providers may be more inclined to self-treat using CAM."[9] In other words, well-educated, more affluent, white female patients are more likely to gravitate toward CAM.

ARE COMPLEMENTARY THERAPIES EFFECTIVE?

The degree to which complementary therapies are effective depends on one's expectations relative to treatment outcomes. If you are engaging in such therapies in an effort to ameliorate tumors that are resistant to standard medical therapies, chances are you will be disappointed by the outcome. However, if your expectations are more modest and focus primarily on improved quality of life, complementary therapies may prove to be of significant value to you. Because quality of life can affect clinical outcomes over time, the value of complementary therapies could be substantial:

> The efficacy of some CAM therapies for cancer treatment and pallia-tion has been documented. Chinese herbal medications are associat-ed with reduced treatment adverse effects, increased quality of life, and improved survival rates across cancer sites. . . . Massage therapy has been shown to reduce lymphedema in breast and gynecologic cancers, and decrease pain and improve mood in patients with ad-vanced cancers. Randomized trials have shown acupuncture reduces the number and severity of hot flashes in women with breast cancer and men with prostate cancer.[10]

Studies have found acupuncture to be useful in managing chemo-therapy-associated vomiting in some cancer patients. Although re-search on acupuncture for cancer pain control and for management of other cancer symptoms is limited, some studies have shown bene-ficial effects that warrant further investigation. A 2008 evidence-based review of clinical options for managing nausea and vomiting in cancer patients noted electroacupuncture as an option to be consid-ered.

Various studies also suggest possible benefits of CAM therapies such as hypnosis, massage, meditation, and yoga in helping cancer patients manage side effects and symptoms of the disease. For exam-ple, a study of 380 patients with advanced cancer concluded that massage therapy may offer some immediate relief for these patients, and that simple touch therapy (placing both hands on specific body sites)—which can be provided by family members and volunteers—may also be helpful. The study was conducted at 15 hospices in the Population-based Palliative Care Research Network.

A 2008 review of the research literature on botanicals and cancer concluded that although several botanicals have shown promise for managing side effects and symptoms such as nausea and vomiting, pain, fatigue, and insomnia, the scientific evidence is limited (the reviewers did not find sufficient evidence to recommend any specific treatment), and many clinical trials have not been well designed. As with use for cancer treatment, use of botanicals for symptom man-agement raises concerns about interactions with cancer drugs, other drugs, and other botanicals.[11]

Clearly, a significant level of research exists demonstrating the effectiveness of selective complementary therapies within the appropriate context. Before engaging in complementary therapies, however, you need to also understand the potential dangers associated with them.

ARE THERE SAFETY ISSUES WITH COMPLEMENTARY OR ALTERNATIVE INTERVENTIONS?

CAM therapies are often marketed as "natural alternatives" to medicine, leading some patients to believe that they are without risks. While prayer, meditation, massage, and other forms of therapy that do not involve the ingestion of any type of compound are generally devoid of risk, other therapies cannot make this claim.

Mary E. advises patients, "If it is something that they ingest, they need to check with the doctors first because it could be counterproductive to treatment."[12] There are three principal dangers when ingesting a diverse range of CAM therapies: (1) There can be a direct reaction to the compounds; (2) The compounds can negatively interact with chemotherapy, radiation therapy, or other medicines; and (3) The CAM compounds/herbals can be contaminated.

CAM products can be very biologically active. In other words,

> Direct adverse effects such as allergic reactions, gastro-intestinal complaints, photosensitivity, skin reactions, and hepatotoxicity [toxic and potentially damaging to the liver] have been reported as side effects to CAM commonly used by cancer patients. For example, Echinacea, used to bolster immunity, has caused allergic reactions including anaphylaxis; St. John's wort, used to treat depression, may cause photosensitivity; black cohosh, used to improve menopausal symptoms, may cause gastrointestinal upset and hepatotoxicity.[13]

The list goes on:

> Drug-supplement interactions have been documented with chemotherapies. St John's wort reduces plasma levels of the active metabolites of three chemotherapy agents: irinotecan, imatinib mesylate, and docetaxel. Acupuncture and intensive manipulative therapies are not advisable in patients with bleeding disorders. Macrobiotic-type diets that limit calorically dense foods may cause cachexia in

some patients. Certain patients also may be at increased risk for rare events associated with massage, including internal hemorrhage, fractures, and infection.[14]

As more and more cancer patients turn to CAM, the number of adverse reactions increases proportionately:

> Side effects and interactions with chemotherapy are being increasingly reported with herb use, and concerns about potential interactions of complementary modalities with biomedical and pharmacologic treatment, safety, efficacy, cost, and establishment of scientific evidence are rising. Given that many botanical supplements lack basic and clinical research documentation and are not closely regulated, many supplements may be contaminated. Toxicity may result from high concentrations of active ingredients in a supplement versus the native form of the natural product. Moreover, there remains a lack of reliable dosage guidelines. Nearly two thirds of individuals reporting use of natural supplements are unaware of drug interactions and information concerning adverse effects, making the assumption that a lack of such information implies safety. Studies on the effects of antioxidants on cancer therapies have yielded mixed results, with some reporting interference, others noting benefits, and most suggesting no significant interaction. Still, caution is recommended for people undergoing treatment with chemotherapy or radiation because it has been proposed that the use of high-dose antioxidants may interfere with the effectiveness of treatment.[15]

If you think these CAM-drug interactions are rare, you are wrong. Researchers state that more than 25 percent of cancer patients who are receiving chemotherapy are likely at risk for a significant adverse reaction.[16] Lori notes:

> When I initially review a patient's medication list, I first make sure they have listed all prescription and nonprescription medications, as well as vitamins, herbs, and supplements. The fish oil they take may be dangerous because it increases their risk of bleeding; the antioxidant vitamin C can potentially interfere with the intended effects of radiation. The soy estrogen may stimulate their breast cancer to grow. In all of these situations, seemingly innocuous supplements can potentially cause harm. My best advice is to not to take any

supplement unless approved by your doctor while undergoing cancer therapies.

As if these dangers were not enough, there are also safety concerns related to the manufacturing processes for CAM products. Many herbal preparations are manufactured in foreign countries with far less stringent manufacturing standards to protect product safety and purity. As a result, so-called *all natural* products may be contaminated with lead, cadmium, arsenic, or other toxins. Even in the United States, oversight of CAM products pales compared to the scrutiny applied to traditional pharmaceutical manufacturing.

The sheer number of herbal remedies marketed makes the challenge of validating their effectiveness, purity, and safety almost Herculean. Dr. Edzard Ernst, emeritus professor at the University of Exeter, makes this point abundantly clear:

> There are about 6,000—that is a really rough estimate—different herbal remedies, and each of them has its own dangers, its own risks. But generally speaking, the risks are, of course, toxicity of the herb itself, and then interactions with prescribed drugs. Here we only know the tip of the iceberg because research into this area has only just begun. We know that herbs have the potential to interact, but we don't know enough about the subject. If we are dealing with Asian herbal mixtures in particular, we know that many of them are contaminated and/or adulterated—adulterated with prescription drugs and contaminated, for instance, with heavy metals, which obviously can cause harm. The biggest danger of all is that these supplements might be used as a true alternative to effective treatments. In this situation, a harmless but ineffective remedy can almost immediately become life-threatening.[17]

QUACKS—IMPOSTERS WHO GIVE COMPLEMENTARY MEDICINE A BAD NAME

Just as it was important to agree on a definition of *CAM*, so, too, should we agree on what constitutes *quackery*: "Quackery is the promotion of false or unproven remedies for profit. This includes any method that has not met the requirements of the United States Food, Drug and Cosmetic Act (FDCA) for either experimental or clinical purposes."[18]

And quackery is commonplace at times when the stakes are high and traditional medicine appears to offer little in the way of a cure: "Cancer patients and their loved ones are wise if they recognize the vulnerability eloquently described by an expert on quackery. In the face of the great leveler, Death, we are all like children listening fearfully for the footsteps of doom, and relieved only by the whisperings of hope. Quacks are peddlers of hope."[19]

There can be a fine line between some forms of CAM and quackery. Quackery in cancer has been around since the disease was first diagnosed. The February 28, 1955, issue of *Time* magazine stated:

> Although U.S. doctors have long known about the damage done by quack cancer cures, they often lack specific clinical evidence to back them up. At a meeting of the International College of Surgeons in Washington last week, Dr. Charles E. Horton of Duke University Hospital produced a sizable body of evidence: 64 case histories of men and women who had first gone to backwoods cancer quacks and then, uncured, had gone on to Duke.[20]

Most medical professionals have an understandable and profound aversion to quacks. Dr. David Gorski, writing for *Science-Based Medicine*, states:

> I despise cancer quacks. It doesn't much matter to me whether the quack is a true believer or a calculating con artist, the end result is the same: People with cancer throwing their one best chance to survive away chasing pixie dust and promises of "natural" cures without the toxicity that is the unfortunate byproduct of the surgery, radiation, and chemotherapy that are the mainstays of our current armamentarium against cancer. I'm a cancer surgeon.[21]

Dr. Gorski goes on to describe a case in which a purported "quack" uses the following attributes to define the cause of a woman's breast cancer:

> The causes of Danielle's breast cancer include, according to Young, rarely drinking water, not eating consistently, eating big meals, eating sugar, not taking deep breaths, being indoors too much, being under stress, being impatient and judgmental, not getting enough sleep, having a "clogged up digestive system" (remember the "toxins" and colon flushes), having blood "full of yeast," and, of course, being

exposed to all sorts of "toxins." It's a veritable cornucopia of nonsensical ideas about human physiology that have little or no (with an emphasis on "no") grounding in science.[22]

I have attended meetings where the virtues of miracle cures were peddled to unsuspecting patients with merciless conviction. And when I challenged these hucksters—demanding valid proof of their claims—I was routed out of the audience with great haste. In one case, a death threat followed. What I found most surprising was the degree to which intelligent, rational individuals were buying into this nonsense. It spoke volumes about their extreme vulnerability and desperate need for hope.

If you think you are immune to the "charms" of a quack, think again. Even the most astute, well-educated patients have fallen prey: "Psychopathic traits of superficial charm and pathological lying, when exhibited by a quack practitioner giving cancer patients the very words they want to hear such as 'cancer cure,' can lead the vulnerable patient into their grasp."[23]

A CASE STUDY IN QUACKERY: THE MAGIC OF ELECTROMAGNETISM

Since the dawn of electricity, people have experimented with ways to harness the power of this energy to heal the human body. Today, some of the most potent diagnostic and treatment modalities, ranging from CT scans to radiation therapy, rely on electromagnetic energy. So, too, do unproven modalities that emit trace levels of electrical current, magnetic fields, or various radio frequencies. Among them is the Rife machine.

The Rife machine was first produced by an American inventor named Royal Raymond Rife. Rife believed that cancer was caused by bacteria that could be destroyed by certain electromagnetic frequencies:

> Rife claimed to have documented a "Mortal Oscillatory Rate" for various pathogenic organisms, and to be able to destroy the organisms by vibrating them at this particular rate. According to the *San Diego Evening Tribune* in 1938, Rife stopped short of claiming that

he could cure cancer, but did argue that he could "devitalize disease organisms" in living tissue, "with certain exceptions."[24]

Rife's beliefs and his device survived him and actually enjoyed a renaissance, thanks to author Barry Lynes and his book *The Cancer Cure That Worked*.[25] Lynes asserts that the Rife machine can cure cancer and that its effectiveness was suppressed by a conspiracy of traditional medical organizations.[26]

What are the incontrovertible facts about the Rife machine? Here are a few to consider:

- The machine has no scientific basis upon which to make outlandish claims.
- The machine is not approved for use in medical treatment by the FDA.
- "Devices bearing Rife's name began to be produced and marketed in the 1980s. Such 'Rife devices' have figured prominently in several cases of health fraud in the U.S., typically centered around the uselessness of the devices and the grandiose claims with which they are marketed."[27]
- "In 2002 John Bryon Krueger, who operated the Royal Rife Research Society, was sentenced to 12 years in prison for his role in a murder and also received a concurrent 30-month sentence for illegally selling Rife devices. In 2009 a U.S. court convicted James Folsom of 26 felony counts for sale of the Rife devices sold as 'NatureTronics,' 'AstroPulse,' 'BioSolutions,' 'Energy Wellness,' and 'Global Wellness.'"[28]

A Google search of the terms *buy Rife machine* turned up more than 1,250,000 responses! So, there's no shortage of vendors willing to sell you an unproven device at significant expense.

QUACKERY IS BIG BUSINESS

Quackery in cancer is more an industry than a chance phenomenon, raking in as much as $4 billion annually, or four times the yearly research budget for the National Cancer Institute; "A widely available compendium lists 78 'treatment centers,' 20 'educational centers,' 41 'support groups,' and 22 'informational services' that promote nonstandard cancer methods. Between 10% and 30% of cancer patients in the United States try quack therapies, and the numbers appear to be considerably higher in other countries."[29]

Patients who fall victim to quackery have many of the same characteristics of CAM patients:

> they have been seduced by claims that the unapproved therapies are "natural" and "non-toxic." Patients who try quack therapies are more likely to be white, female, foreign born, and above average in education and income. More important are a person's attitudes. Victims are more likely to believe that their cancers could have been prevented through stress reduction, diet, and environmental factors; that disease in general is caused mainly by poor nutrition, stress and worry; that standard therapies are useless or harmful; and, that unorthodox remedies are beneficial.[30]

THE DANGERS OF QUACKERY

Like alternative medicines, cancer quackery can take a toll that far exceeds the cost paid by patients: "The great tragedy of cancer quackery is that patients needlessly die as a result of being diverted from effective standard treatment."[31]

Cancer quacks exploit the gambler's fallacy, the erroneous notion that there is "nothing to lose" by trying dubious remedies. In fact, the threats of questionable therapies include:

- **Incompetent Practitioners.** Quack cancer treatments, including some which have involved the use of improperly applied legitimate methods, have maimed or killed cancer patients. Examples include brain damage caused by misusing whole body hyperthermia, toxic overdoses of chemotherapy, caustic chemicals applied externally, poisonous herbal compounds, and improperly performed surgery. Cancer patients treated by incompetent practitioners lose out on two scales as both therapeutic risks increase and potential benefits decrease.
- **Hazardous Clinical Conditions.** Cancer patients have been infected by contaminated medications, developed septicemia fol-

lowing perforations of their colons during insertion of enema devices, and acquired infections from unsterile needles.

- **Interfering with Proper Clinical Management.** Patients who try to "cover all bases" by mixing conventional and questionable treatments may diminish the effectiveness of their medications by ingesting megadoses of vitamins or minerals, or having injections of unusual chemicals.[32]

SOURCES OF TRUSTWORTHY INFORMATION

Complementary therapies can have a profoundly positive impact on cancer patients when expectations are appropriate and the therapies are properly utilized. There are numerous sources of trusted information that you may wish to consider before engaging in complementary therapies, including:

- The American Cancer Society: http://www.cancer.org/treatment/ treatmentsandsideeffects/complementaryandalternativemedicine/ index
- National Cancer Institute's Office of Cancer Complementary and Alternative Medicine (OCCAM): http://cam.cancer.gov/cam
- National Institutes of Health's National Center for Complementary and Alternative Medicine (NCCAM): http://nccam.nih.gov.

DISCUSSING COMPLEMENTARY AND ALTERNATIVE THERAPIES WITH YOUR PHYSICIAN

It's important that you feel comfortable discussing complementary medicine with your physicians. Research indicates that the "majority of CAM use is not being communicated to providers."[33] Because we have seen how certain CAM therapies can interact with traditional treatment modalities or cause harm in other ways, this reluctance to share such information with your physicians must be overcome. Only then are you in a truly collaborative partnership with your doctor.

14

THE ROLE OF YOUR CAREGIVERS

Dana B. is apprehensive by nature. As she puts it, "My entire life, I've been a worrier."[1] So the prospect of facing stage 3 breast cancer was particularly daunting for the fifth-grade teacher, wife, and mother of two daughters. Fortunately, Dana had a strong group of caregivers who accompanied her to the treatment, held her hand, shopped for groceries, and provided support in innumerable other ways:

> My husband was incredibly supportive. He was always there with a shoulder to cry on, and he held my hand a lot! He picked up a ton of household duties that I would otherwise have done. He stepped into a role and did it with ease.
>
> I had incredibly supportive friends who also stepped up and did anything I needed. They had meals delivered all of the time! For me, keeping up a so-called normal life relative to my work helped immensely. Simply being around kids and going on with my normal routine was amazingly therapeutic![2]

At this point in our interview, Dana stopped for a moment, looked down, and then slowly raised her chin, her eyes brimming with tears:

> My tears are not about me having cancer but about the compassion that was poured out upon me by friends, colleagues, and family. One of the most touching experiences I had was at school.
>
> I had told my students only the basic facts that I felt they needed to know: I had breast cancer and that, when they came back from

winter break, I would have a wig on because I would lose my hair due to chemotherapy.

When I came back from winter break with my new wig, two boys showed up with shaved heads. That started a whole rally of kids supporting me, from the boys shaving their heads to the girls putting pink streaks in their hair. They had fundraisers and donated the money raised to the Susan B. Komen Foundation.

There were times when I would just take a moment to look around and realize that God was working in all directions.[3]

Many cancer patients like Dana are blessed to have a circle of family and friends eager to help them address the many challenges that arise during the journey through cancer. Within this circle, it can be beneficial to have one or two individuals who will be present throughout the course of your treatment. That way, you have an individual who has heard all of the important information provided by your physicians and has observed your treatment. This person can be a spouse, adult child, sibling, or close friend.

The demands on your caregiver can be quite high, and it is essential you and your caregiver understand and agree on the responsibilities of the role in advance. That way there is less opportunity for feelings of disappointment or a sense of unanticipated burden.

COMMON RESPONSIBILITIES FOR THE CAREGIVER

Your caregiver will help address your physical and emotional needs and act as your advocate with health care providers. The American Cancer Society (ACS) provides a good outline of some typical caregiver responsibilities. Here's a short list of ways that your caregiver can assist you with daily living:

- Grocery shopping and meal preparation
- Assistance with eating
- Ensure that you take your medications as scheduled
- Assist with bathing, grooming, and dressing
- Help with toileting
- Maintain the home and laundry
- Stay current on bills

- Ensure that your emotional needs are being met
- Provide transportation for medical appointments
- Respond to emerging medical needs when you are at home
- When new issues arise, decide whether they warrant medical attention. [4]

Diane C.'s caregiver was her husband, Rick. As Diane puts it, "The caregiver has the toughest job. They are juggling all of the balls in the real world. Rick took care of the household. Rick paid all of the bills. He was also there to be positive for me. He just made life bearable. I wasn't a patient to him. When it was scary, he was there." [5]

Diane adds that Rick's job was made even more complicated by the fact that "We had just closed on our new house two days before I was diagnosed, and we had planned to redo it completely." [6]

Your caregiver also provides invaluable assistance when you interface with the medical community. He or she can help you prepare in advance for doctors' visits so you get optimal value from each clinic appointment.

Because many physicians allocate only so much time for each appointment, the ACS advises the caregiver:

> Work with the patient before you go to figure out the most important things you need to talk about. Make a list of questions and concerns. For instance, what symptoms do you need to tell the cancer team about? When did they start? Making a list ahead of time to take with you will help you to use your time in the office well. And it means you won't forget anything important. [7]

Even if the doctor seems a bit pressed, the ACS advises, "Don't leave the office until your doctor answers all your questions and you both understand what to do next. Nurses can also be great sources of information, and you might get to spend more time with them than the doctor." [8] We are all respectful of the pressures on today's physicians, but as Lori will tell you, those pressures come with the job.

From Lori's perspective, it helps immensely when the patient and caregiver are organized when presenting the patient's symptoms and questions:

This helps us use our time together wisely, as there is so much to cover. Sometimes we cannot address everything during one appointment. Therefore, I ask my patients to prioritize their concerns. If we run out of time, we set a new appointment to complete the task. The caregiver can really help by being a scribe and accurately sharing the discussion with the patient and other family members after the appointment. It is also immensely helpful to the physician to have a primary point of contact who can represent the interests of the broader family.

Your caregiver can be an active listener and scribe at each appointment. Because your thinking may not be as clear as normal nor your memory as good, your caregiver can step in to help. He or she can then act as an independent source of information to verify that your "take-aways" from conversations with physicians are accurate.

Another important role relates to medications. When you receive a new prescription, your caregiver can help ensure that you understand what you are being given and why. They can also ask:

- How frequently is the medication to be taken and in what dosage?
- Can it be taken on an empty stomach, or should it be taken with food or water? Are there foods or supplements to be avoided when taking this medication?
- What are the potential side effects commonly associated with the medication?
- Can the medication interact with any existing drug you are on?
- Is the cost of the medication covered by insurance, and what is your potential out-of-pocket cost for it?
- If prohibitively expensive, is there a less expensive, therapeutically effective alternative?

The ACS reminds patients to "Be sure you add this medicine to the list of all the medicines the patient is taking."[9]

All of these new responsibilities can cause significant strain in a caregiver who has had little preparation for managing the impact of cancer and its treatment on a loved one. Though they may act with grace, stress can also undermine their well-being:

Even though family caregivers are the long-term care providers to people with cancer, they receive little preparation, information, or support to carry out their vital role. Family caregivers often are expected to navigate an increasingly complex and fragmented health care system on their own and to find whatever help that may be available. In recent years, the caregiving responsibilities of family members have increased dramatically, primarily due to the use of toxic treatments in outpatient settings, the decline in available health care resources, and the shortage of health care providers. Family caregivers of cancer patients have participated in a limited number of intervention programs but these programs have focused almost exclusively on improving patient outcomes (e.g., symptom management, quality of life) with less attention directed to the needs of family caregivers.[10]

THE CAREGIVER'S NEED TO HAVE THE PATIENT'S CONSENT

For your caregiver to be most effective, they must be privy to the confidential information shared with you by your physicians. Privacy laws in the United States stringently regulate how and when medical information can be disclosed. Therefore, your caregiver must have formal, written consent from you acknowledging their right to receive privileged health care information regarding your diagnosis, treatment, and status:

The simplest and most common way is for the patient to fill out a release form that allows the doctor to discuss their care with you. Talk to the doctor about what steps need to be taken so that the health care team can discuss the patient's care with you. Then be sure that there's a copy in the patient's records and keep the release form up to date. It's also a good idea to keep a backup copy for your files. When you call the doctor's office, you may need to remind them that they have the form and they can discuss the patient's care with you.[11]

CARING FOR THE CAREGIVER

As both a patient and later a caregiver, Diane C. states, "I would also tell caregivers to take care of themselves. They are going to be burning the candle at both ends, and I don't think they know how tiring it becomes."[12]

Caregivers suffer in many of the same ways that cancer patients do. In fact, research has shown that caregivers often mirror the emotional states of the loved ones for whom they care. Cancer patients and their family caregivers react to cancer as one emotional system; there is a significant reciprocal relationship between each person's response to the illness, with family caregivers often reporting as much emotional distress, anxiety, or depression as patients. The advanced phase of cancer is especially difficult for family caregivers, who sometimes report more depression than patients themselves. However, caregivers seldom use any form of mental health services to deal with their own depression or emotional distress, and this puts them at risk for long-term health problems.[13]

None of this should come as a surprise when you realize that, from the caregiver's perspective, "Suddenly you've been asked to care for the person with cancer, and you are also needed to help make decisions about medical care and treatment. None of this is easy. There will be times when you know you've done well, and times when you just want to give up. This is normal."[14]

Darrell H. related a memory from the time when Patricia began her twenty-year odyssey with lymphoma: "One memory I have is of a day when Patricia needed to go to the clinic for treatment. I took the day off from work to watch the kids. I watched Patricia drive off, and I just stood there in the living room and burst into tears. How am I going to take care of these two kids? God, this is awful."[15]

According to an article in *CA: A Cancer Journal for Clinicians*,

> There are many causes of stress and distress in cancer caregivers. Dealing with the crisis of cancer in someone you love, the uncertain future that lies ahead, financial worries, difficult decisions that must be made, and unexpected and unwanted lifestyle changes are just a few of them. Fear, hopelessness, guilt, confusion, doubt, anger, and helplessness can take a toll on both the person with cancer and the

caregiver. And while the focus tends to be on the patient, all of this affects the physical and mental health of the caregiver, too.[16]

Just as stress and distress can lead to depression and anxiety in cancer patients, it can it also impede the well-being of caregivers. In fact, depression is relatively common among caregivers. The ACS advises,

> Everyone has emotional ups and downs, but if a person always feels down, has no energy, cries a lot, or is easily angered, it may be a warning sign of depression. Many people see the feelings of depression as a sign of weakness rather than a sign that something is out of balance, but ignoring or denying these feelings will not make them go away. Early attention to symptoms of depression can make a big difference in how the caregiver feels about their role and how well they can do the things they need to do.[17]

It is not just emotional issues that cause caregivers to struggle. Their physical health, over time, can also be affected by the demands of caring for a seriously ill loved one. As a result, they often pay little attention to their own needs to rest, exercise, or get medical care. This issue can be particularly problematic for older caregivers who suffer from various chronic conditions.[18]

SOMETHING TO SHARE WITH YOUR PHYSICIAN

Until recently, the needs of the caregiver have been largely ignored by the medical community. Clinicians need to recognize that patients and their family caregivers react to cancer as a unit, and as a result, they both have legitimate needs for help from health professionals. There is general consensus in the literature that, when patients and caregivers are treated simultaneously, important synergies are achieved that contribute to the well-being of each person. When caregivers' needs are not addressed, their mental and physical health is at risk, and patients are denied the opportunity to obtain optimal care from a well-prepared family caregiver.[19]

DON'T KEEP SECRETS

One way to help minimize problems for both the caregiver and patient is by ensuring open, honest, and frequent communication: "Problems occur when patients and caregivers hide worries from one another, and avoid talking about sensitive issues associated with cancer and its treatments."[20] Communication may help both you and your caregiver work through troubling issues, forging an even stronger bond between the two of you.

Parents often struggle with whether to keep things secret from their children. Dana B. was no exception, struggling with what to share openly with her children: "I think one fault of mine is that I have not been very open with them. I don't show my emotions around them. I try to protect them just as my husband tries to protect me. I don't always think this is healthy. I've learned over time that it is okay for them to see me cry and for them to know that this is difficult. It helps them see that they need to express their emotions."[21]

ASK OTHERS TO PITCH IN

Your caregiver needs and deserves a break. They also deserve acknowledgment of the hard work they are doing and the difficult emotional time they may be managing. Other members of your family, as well as your friends, can be extremely helpful by:

- offering to help with some of the daily tasks of living—from shopping to cleaning to childcare,
- giving the caregiver a day off from attending one of your medical treatments,
- listening and validating their struggles and concerns so that they feel cared for as well, and
- keeping your circle of family and friends informed about your health status.[22]

A PATIENT'S ADVICE FOR A CAREGIVER

Shelley W. offers some straightforward and solid advice for caregivers based on her and her husband's journey:

> If you see a role you can fill during the process that is based on your strengths, then do that. Keep the lines of communication open for discussing feelings and duties throughout treatment. Seek resources and/or support groups for caregivers if you are interested in talking with other caregivers about their experiences. Acknowledge that your feelings about the journey are important, too.[23]

ADVICE FOR PATIENTS

"This journey involves others. It is not just about you," says Myra C. Myra describes herself as private person who felt challenged by the outpouring of caring offerings from friends. She learned an important lesson through the process of managing this challenge to her privacy:

> Our friends wanted to bring dinner or help clean the house. I'm a really private person and felt that we didn't need this type of help. My daughter said to me, "Mom, this is not about you. It's about them. They need to be able to show they care. All you have to do is say 'Thank you.'" We were always the ones who did for others. It was good for us to learn how to say "Thank you."[24]

Lori offers advice from the perspective of patient, caregiver, and physician:

> I remember a time when I was caring for my mother. She was clearly just a few weeks away from dying of ovarian cancer. As the oncologist in the family, I felt a medical responsibility, and as her daughter, I desperately wanted to hold on to those last days. I had not been back home to Kansas City in a month and was feeling so fatigued! My husband and siblings all offered to help; I just didn't want to accept it. But once I decided to take a few days and go home, it helped so much to refresh and reenergize me so that I could face the days ahead. It became clear that I had to take care of myself and also accept the help of others.

This lesson was repeated when I was first diagnosed with breast cancer. I was hesitant to share my situation with more than a very small inner circle of family and friends. I did not want to be a person labeled by my cancer. But once I realized that part of healing is allowing others in—to bring a meal, weed our garden, offer encouragement through a card or e-mail, or pray for me—it became part of my healing process. It opened me up to share with others, including my patients. As a person who never needed anyone's help, it felt really good to allow people in.

III

After Initial Treatments Are Over

15

WHEN INITIAL TREATMENT PROVES INSUFFICIENT

"Cancer is not a straight line. It's up and down."[1]

—Elizabeth Edwards

Within a few weeks of our meeting with Dr. M., Lori was scheduled for surgery. Based on her initial testing, Lori chose to undergo a lumpectomy, otherwise known as breast-conserving therapy (BCT).

The morning of Lori's surgery began with a procedure designed to help identify Lori's sentinel nodes (the specific lymph nodes under her arm where fluid draining from the affected area of her breast naturally collected). The sentinel nodes would be biopsied to ensure that they did not harbor cancerous cells. It would be an important part of Lori's final staging; once cancerous cells from the primary tumor enter the lymphatic system, they can be transported to other parts of the body, allowing the potential development of additional tumors, or metastases, over time.

Radioactive dye was injected into the area of Lori's tumor. After an appropriate amount of time had elapsed, a nuclear imaging technician began tracing the pathway of the dye as it gradually flowed from her breast into her lymphatic system. This process would provide the surgeon with a roadmap to identify which nodes to remove. The sentinel nodes would be examined by a pathologist during surgery. If cancerous cells were identified, additional nodes would be sampled. This process would continue until the nodes that were excised showed no signs of cancer.

Our next move was to the preoperative, or surgical holding, area, where we would await Dr. M. Nurses reviewed Lori's medical history, took her vital signs, started her IV, and asked her to reconfirm, in her own words, the nature of the procedure she was about to undergo. This process is medicine's equivalent of a preflight check, designed to reduce the likelihood of errors.

Dr. M. arrived shortly thereafter and told us that all lights were green for Lori's procedure. The nurse anesthetist filled a small syringe with Versed, a potent amnesic. Before injecting it into Lori's IV line, the nurse anesthetist suggested I say my goodbyes now, while Lori's memory was still intact. I would see her in recovery following surgery.

Squeezing my wife's hand and looking deeply into her beautiful eyes, I said, "I love you with all of my heart, and I'll be praying that everything goes perfectly."

We kissed, and then Lori was on her way to the OR.

It's hard to sit still while waiting for someone you love to emerge from surgery. Although it was only a few hours, the time passed incredibly slowly. As I looked around the waiting area, I saw a half-dozen families patiently biding their time. Some were reading months-old magazines, while others half-listened to Oprah on the television. Like Lori, their loved ones lay motionless in a nearby OR, their fate in the hands of surgeons, as well as in the hands of God. I prayed that everyone would be okay.

Three hours passed before Dr. M. met me in the waiting room. The smile on his face more than hinted that good news would follow: "Lori did great. She's in the first stage of recovery, and you'll be able to see her in an hour or two. The tumor was pretty much what we expected, and I believe we got it all. The early path reports indicate that her sentinel nodes are clear. It's all great news, John!"

My eyes welled up in relief, knowing that Lori was going to be okay. "Thank you so much" was about all I could muster.

Before departing, Dr. M. reminded me that we needed to wait a few days for the final pathology report confirming that the margins were, indeed, clear. He was referring to the area of normal tissue surrounding the tumor. Clear margins indicate that the healthy tissue has not been infiltrated by cancer cells and the surgeon has removed all signs of disease from the affected area.

It was not long before I was again holding my precious wife's hand and telling her the good news. Nor was it long before we were able to depart St. Joseph Medical Center for home.

As Lori states:

> My recovery was amazingly smooth and fast. I was up and around the next day, organizing and packing for our upcoming move to our new home in two weeks. My energy bounced right back, and I essentially had no pain. One of my first questions was, "When can I resume exercise?" Though relieved by the early report of favorable findings, I knew enough to remain cautiously optimistic until the pathology report was finalized.
>
> Two days later, just as I was getting ready to sit down to lunch, Dr. V. called with the pathology. Dr. V. is a friend and a colleague, so I immediately sensed by her tone of voice that the news was not going to be good. She dreaded telling me my findings: that the margins were not clear and, in fact, tumor cells infiltrated numerous surgical margins, meaning that cancer appeared to have invaded a larger area of my breast than detected during my own exam, the diagnostic imaging, and surgery.
>
> Dr. V. was sending tissue samples from the tumor for additional genetic analysis. That would provide some insight into the relative aggressiveness of the cancer, as well as the probability of a recurrence and need for chemotherapy. I could hear my own voice quivering as I asked her specific questions. Once again, just like the night I first discovered the lump, I felt kicked in the stomach—sad, fearful, anxious, and disappointed. My hope for minimal surgery was over, and I would need to go back for more. This meant mastectomy as well as reconstruction, surgery that is far more extensive than originally planned. But I had seen so many of my patients go through it, and that, along with my faith, gave me great comfort that it would be okay.

WHEN AN INITIAL TREATMENT PROVES INSUFFICIENT

Cancer treatments fail. It's that simple. Though patients enter treatment with great hope, that hope may be dashed when either further evidence of disease or proof of recurrence is discovered. Sometimes the failure is apparent immediately, as was the case with Lori's lumpectomy. Other times the disease reappears months, years, even decades later. It is not always easy to evaluate the effectiveness of your cancer treatment.

The effectiveness of surgery is often defined by the surgeon's ability to completely remove the tumor. The clearance around the tumor is referred to as the *margin*. This term indicates that, upon microscopic evaluation of the tissue adjacent to the tumor, there is no evidence of residual cancer cells. If a surgeon is unable to achieve clear margins, additional surgery or other forms of treatment will likely be required. Even with clear margins, additional treatment designed to prevent a recurrence may be initiated, such as radiation or chemotherapy. This is known by the term *adjuvant therapy*.

The effectiveness of nonsurgical treatments, such as radiation therapy and chemotherapy, is often measured using physical exams, lab tests, and diagnostic imaging techniques, often referred to as *scans*. Two commonly performed scans are CT and PET, which are discussed in chapter 1. PET scans can help illuminate ongoing metabolic activity in tumors, showing whether a tumor is still functioning or biologically active. CT scans can reveal the degree to which a tumor is shrinking or continuing to grow. These tests not only reveal whether treatment is effectively diminishing the primary tumor but can also determine if the cancer has metastasized to other parts of the body.

Evidence of ongoing cancer can be seen in an analysis of a patient's blood. For hematologic cancers, such as leukemia, blood analyses are immediately revelatory regarding the patient's condition. But blood tests can also tell a great deal about solid tumors, such as ovarian cancer and prostate cancer, by measuring certain indicators, known as "markers," that fluctuate with tumor activity.

In addition to testing, regular physical exams by your health care provider are an important means of establishing whether your disease is active. The frequency of testing will vary based on (1) the nature of one's disease; (2) the ability for a scan or blood test to yield meaningful information; (3) the beliefs and practices of one's physician; and (4) the patient's compliance, particularly once they have been deemed a cancer "survivor."

Whether treatment success is measured by a surgical pathology report, scan, exam, or blood test, a patient might find that testing rekindles much of the anxiety experienced at the time of the initial diagnosis. So much is riding on the results. The results can be either reassuring or, in some cases, devastating. No one wants to learn that the difficult treatment they have endured has proven ineffective or that a remission appears to have ended; nor does any physician relish sharing such difficult news.

As Lori states,

> One of the most difficult moments for me as a physician is delivering bad news. Patients and their loved ones have often endured much anguish during treatment in the hope of a positive outcome. You can see it in their eyes—a fragile sense of hope that can be dashed with the revelation of new test results. We are taught in medical school how to plan and deliver treatments but not how to soften the blow when the news is hard. After twenty-five years, it is still among the hardest things I do.

HITTING THE RESET BUTTON

If your initial treatment failed to cure your cancer, then you have reached another crucial signpost along your journey: the need to modify your treatment plan to include new modalities of care. It's a bit like hitting the reset button and starting the game over. This can be a particularly difficult time for many patients because the preferred treatment option has proven unsuccessful, often triggering new waves of anxiety and doubt.

When Diane C. learned that she was conquering leukemia, a huge load was lifted from her shoulders. However, the relief was to prove only temporary. Soon a new load was added—her husband, Rick, was desperately ill. Diane recounts:

> It started with a pea-sized cyst on the back of Rick's neck. He didn't say a word about it. He watched it for about six months. Then one day I hugged him just right, putting my hand on the back of his head, and felt this golf-ball-sized cyst. I jumped about three feet and said, "What's that!" Rick said that his PCP told him it was "old-man's fatty

tissue disease," and they were watching it. I said, "Oh really. How long has this been going on?" I told him we were going to see a surgeon.

Dr. M. took it out and thought it was nothing to worry about. He was confident that he had gotten it all. They sent it to pathology, and it came back stage 4 melanoma. When we went and got the results, everyone was shocked. Dr. M. said, "I know that I should have gotten more surrounding tissue, but I never would have guessed that it was melanoma." He advised us to see an oncologist.

The oncologist suggested that we go to MD Anderson, which we did. The doctors at MD Anderson told us that they could not help us because, at the time, Rick appeared to be cancer free. They did scans, examined him head to toe, and they couldn't find anything.

Two months later, Rick doubled over in pain in a parking lot. He came home and waited for me to come home from work. When I came home, he said, "I think I need to go to the emergency room."

We're thinking, "Maybe this is an appendicitis." The ER doctor said, "I've got really bad news. Your adrenal gland has burst. It is the cancer, and it is everywhere." We were stunned.

At that point we were worried that we might not get Rick home. They admitted him. Dr. B. saw him. She came in and said, "I don't know what we are going to do for you, but now that you have clearly defined tumors, you can go back to MD Anderson. You are going to be okay. You are going to beat this." She gave him that pep talk, saying, "It's not the end of the road, but the beginning of the road for you."

He was on a clinical trial for the systemic cancer while also receiving whole-brain radiation plus gamma-knife for brain cancer. Dr. B. told Rick he could go out fighting or just go out. He fought. Rick fought like hell. I thought, if I bought into it, we were going to lose. I wasn't delusional—the diagnosis was terminal—but when is the expiration date? I had been "terminal," and I'm sitting here seven years after treatment talking to you. So miracles do happen.[2]

Rick's disease progressed mercilessly fast, as happens with certain types of cancers, such as metastatic melanoma. By contrast, other people have diseases that are far more indolent. They may experience multiple remissions followed by setbacks, followed by changes in therapy—all in the hope of staving off the cancer. Patricia H. was to repeat this cycle many times over twenty years, as can be seen in Darrell's recollection about the end of the first remission:

When the diagnosis was confirmed [in 1993], she went to Dr. J., who gave her CHOP [a standard four-drug chemotherapy regimen for lymphoma]. It worked, and Patricia had an eight-year remission. In fact, there was a time in 2000 when, at a checkup, the doctors said, "Wow! We may have beaten this thing." Once the remission happened, we thought we may have indeed beaten the odds.

Then, six months later, she had a recurrence. My initial feeling was, "OK. Let's treat it again." I didn't understand that you could not simply repeat the same treatment. I thought, "Let's just bring out the CHOP. It worked for eight years, so let's do it again." But it doesn't work that way.

The first treatment they tried didn't work. Then the doctor said, "This might be hairy-cell leukemia, which is different than lymphoma. Let's try this treatment for hairy-cell leukemia."

About this time, Patricia heard an NPR story about Rituxan, so she said, "Wait a minute. What about this drug I heard about called Rituxan?" The doctor said he didn't think Patricia was a great candidate for it and that it probably wouldn't work on her. So he gave her the treatment for hairy-cell leukemia, which failed.

We are getting to a point where her symptoms are worsening. She is developing pain in her back from a small tumor developing along her spine. Two therapies haven't worked. So, all of a sudden, it's getting pretty rough. She's losing weight and feeling miserable.

I remember sitting with her in the exam room when she said to the doctor, "Look, I'm so miserable. What happens if we just don't do anything else?" He says, "Well, you probably have weeks left."

It was at that point he said, "I think we need to try Rituxan because anything else will probably kill you. You are so weak that all the other therapies are not good options." Rituxan had only been approved for about eighteen months. I picked up a pamphlet on it and read that it only works for about one in two patients. The thought that formed in my head was that we were down to a coin flip.

By the time she came out after a second treatment, I thought, "Wow. This is working." I could see her changing. There was a period of recuperation. She was thin as a rail, but she built her strength back up over the next year. This remission lasted until November 2004.[3]

THE "MIDDLE STAGE" OF CANCER

Many patients enter a midpoint in their journey with cancer. It is what author and ovarian cancer survivor Susan Gubar defines as the "middle stage." Writing in a June 5, 2014, article in the *New York Times*, Gubar stated:

> For some of us, there is a middle stage in this journey. Because of advances in cancer research and the efforts of dedicated oncologists, a large population today deals with disease kept in abeyance. The cancer has returned and has been controlled, but it will never go away completely. Like me, these people cope with cancer that is treatable for some unforeseeable amount of time. Chronic cancer means you will die from it—unless you are first hit by the proverbial bus—but not now, not necessarily soon.
>
> The word "chronic" resides between the category of cured and the category of terminal. It refers to disease that is not spreading, malignancy that can be arrested but not eradicated. At times, the term may seem incommensurate with repetitive and arduous regimens aimed at an (eventually) fatal disease. For unlike diabetes or asthma, cancer does not respond predictably to treatment.
>
> Still, quite a few patients with some types of leukemia or lymphoma, prostate or ovarian cancer live for years. While in the 1970s, 10 percent of women with metastatic breast cancer survived five or more years, today up to 40 percent do. Chronic disease may lack the drama of diagnosis and early treatment; even friends can get bored by mounting details. Its evolution does not conform to the feel-good stories of recovery that most of us want to read. But neither does it adhere to the frightfully degenerative plot of quickly advancing tumors.[4]

PATRICIA'S ONGOING SAGA

Patricia lived a long time in that middle stage. She would have to endure far more interventions over the decade that followed her treatment with Rituxan:

> In 2004, a tumor broke Patricia's leg. I was officiating at our son's wedding in our backyard, when Patricia tried to push something out

of the way with her left foot. She let out a small cry of pain. So she sat in a chair through the ceremony and pictures that followed. She was a trooper. She was a tough cookie! I helped her to bed later that night and took her to the ER the next morning. They said a tumor had caused a spiral fracture of the bone, and she needed surgery.

Dr. R. did the surgery. We loved him. He joked with us. He said, "I have it so much easier than the medical oncologists. When I see something bad, I just cut it out. They have to give you poison!"

When she was recovering, the doctors said that her lymphoma had transformed into a much more aggressive, large-cell lymphoma, so they sent us to see Dr. S. at Saint Luke's. He told Patricia that she needed a stem cell transplant "yesterday." It was an autologous transplant. We went into the American Cancer Society Hope House and lived there for a month during her treatment. (She needed to be away from family that might infect her.)

Roughly a year to a year and half later she went in for a check, and they found lymphoma cells. The impact on me was to think, "This is it. It's a death sentence." I thought, "If the transplant doesn't do it, you're toast." I took it pretty hard. But the clinic people said, "We have this drug called Gemzar." So they gave her the Gemzar treatments, and about a year later they gave her the all-clear again.[5]

ALLOWING FOR DISAPPOINTMENT WHILE NOT RELINQUISHING HOPE

When you hit these milestones, it is time to be kind to yourself, a time to express your disappointment without relinquishing your hope. You will be traversing a new path on your journey, but first you must understand how the additional knowledge acquired to date about your condition impacts your staging, prognosis, and recommended treatment options. Your physician should provide this information as well as recommended modifications to the treatment plan.

Now's the time to take out your compass and reassess the direction you are headed. It is essential that you go through an appropriate level of due diligence with your doctor regarding the next phase(s) of treatment. Just as you inquired about efficacy, side effects, treatment duration, and other factors prior to your first course of treatment, you need to repeat the process again now. Three very important questions to consider are:

1. What are the goals of this treatment?
2. What is the likelihood it will be successful? and
3. What short-term and long-term effects could the treatment have on my quality of life?

Only after you've completed this process can you truly provide your physician with informed consent to proceed.

EXPANDING THE RANGE OF CLINICAL RESOURCES

Additional physicians may join the team to help you on your journey, depending on the type of treatment(s) being recommended. Whereas you initially could have been treated only by a surgeon, you may now want to consult with a radiation oncologist, medical oncologist, or other specialists. These physicians may be providing simultaneous interventions. It is essential that they be functioning as a well-coordinated team because the administration of one therapeutic regimen could affect the timing, dose, or even usage of another treatment modality. For example, patients undergoing chemotherapy may have to carefully sequence their radiation treatments so they do not overwhelm their bodies and increase the probability of adverse effects.

The stakes are higher now because the first line of medical defense has failed. The chances of having a sustained response to treatment diminish, while the level of risks, side effects, and long-term consequences of therapy may be increased.

DUE DILIGENCE DÉJÀ VU

Just as you asked many questions about your initial treatment, so, too, must you feel fully informed about the next steps in your journey. In addition to understanding the fundamental nature of the recommended treatment, you may also wish to ask your physicians the following questions:

- Why might this treatment be effective when others have failed?
- Are there other options for treatment that we should discuss?

- What are the side effects or after-effects of treatment that I could experience?
- Who will perform this treatment, and what are his or her qualifications for doing so?
- Will my insurance cover the cost of this treatment?
- Where can I learn more about this treatment before agreeing to it?
- What happens if I elect not to have further treatment?

It may be helpful to take a few days, do your own research, talk with your caregiver, and then come to the most informed decision possible. Regardless of the outcome, you will feel as though you entered this phase of treatment with a solid understanding of its probable outcome, side effects, and costs.

REEVALUATING CLINICAL TRIALS

Though clinical trials may not have been appropriate as an initial line of therapy, they could be appropriate now. Ask your physician whether consideration should be given to clinical trials. Your physician can help you answer these questions:

- Are there available trials for your condition and stage of disease?
- Do you meet the eligibility requirements for participation in the trial?
- What would be required of you for participation?
- Will your insurance cover the costs associated with the trial (including not simply the treatment but also ancillary diagnostic services, which can prove costly)?
- What are the risks and the potential benefits of the trial?
- Are there equally good alternatives to the trial?
- What options would remain if the trial treatment proved ineffective in controlling your cancer?

THE END OF ACTIVE TREATMENT FOR LORI

Lori endured a second major surgery—bilateral mastectomies. The difficulty of the recovery was far more than Lori or I anticipated. In Lori's words:

> Once I had a chance to digest the news about my initial pathology, I knew I needed more surgery—a mastectomy. I also knew that my type of cancer was more likely to be present in the opposite breast and to evade early detection by imaging, so I opted for bilateral mastectomies. It would take coordination between my breast surgeon and my reconstructive surgeon, which even under the most optimal circumstances can take several weeks. I decided to allow myself my hour of sadness but then take that energy, become my own advocate, and push hard to get things done as soon as possible.
>
> While waiting for my second surgery, I knew I needed to take care of my spiritual, psychological, and physical needs. I packed much of our house to get ready to move, took time to exercise, read my Bible, and talk to friends. Mother's Day was during that time, and all I wanted was to see my sons, so my husband arranged for them to fly home from California and Wisconsin for the weekend. We talked, went to church, and even took in a baseball game. My surgery was scheduled for early the next week.
>
> The day of surgery was also the day before our scheduled move. My sister Janet, a nurse at Duke University Medical Center, came the night of surgery to help with my care and allow John to be with the movers the next day. She stayed with me those first few days when I felt so physically helpless. She brought me "home" to our new house (and new beginning for me), where we were greeted by a chaotic setting as John worked hard to supervise the movers on a ninety-degree day. Janet's calming presence, encouragement, and hands-on care were invaluable. I will always be grateful she was there by my side. My brother Chris and his wife, Gail, took the second watch and stayed for several days, helping me as I struggled to gain strength as well as helping John unpack our new house. They all dropped their jobs, families, and plans to come and help. Having my strong support system was a tremendous blessing, and I believe it was a key to my recovery.
>
> The final pathology report came out. I held my breath, said a prayer for strength, and waited on the other end of the phone while Dr. V. read me her findings. There proved to be many areas of

cancer creeping through my breast. That was the scary news. But this time there was excellent clearance around the tumor—the margins were negative! A genetic test done to predict my recurrence was also low, so I was not going to need chemotherapy. My risk could be reduced by taking a pill each day to block estrogen.

I knew I had found a silver lining—and a new beginning. Three weeks later I was back at work, now armed with a personal story to complement those of my patients. We would help one another on this journey.

16

THE CHALLENGES OF SURVIVING CANCER

Upon completing treatment and regaining his strength, Bill E. reclaimed his "old world" with a vengeance. He was not about to let cancer rob him of one more precious moment of the retirement he had worked so hard to enjoy. But not everyone responds like Bill.

For Dana B., surviving her initial course of treatment brought its own challenges:

> Post-treatment, I've felt more depressed! I think it's because, during treatment, we were actively doing something to get rid of the cancer. We had a plan. We could stick to the plan, and that relieved my anxiety.
>
> Then, when I was finally out of the treatment phase, something odd happened. You would think that I would be extremely excited and elated that there were no more treatments in front of me. But at the same time, there was a feeling of "Oh, now what? I am on my own!" One minute you are actively doing something to prevent the cancer from coming back, and then all of sudden you are not. [1]

Each person responds in his or her own way to being a cancer survivor:

> You can be a victim of cancer, or a survivor of cancer. It's a mindset. [2]
>
> —Dave Pelzer

Cancer taught me to stop saving things for a special occasion. Every day is special. You don't have to get cancer to start living life to the fullest. My post-cancer philosophy? No wasted time. No ugly clothes. No boring movies.[3]

—Regina Brett

Having had cancer, one important thing to know is you're still the same person at the end. You're stripped down to near zero. But most people come out the other end feeling more like themselves than ever before.[4]

—Kylie Minogue

For those of us who have not made the journey through cancer, there is an irony to the notion of survivorship being a challenge. After all, is this not the answer to our prayers? Yet, those who have completed the journey, the cancer survivors, often discover that, while medicine may have made great strides in treating cancer, they still have much to learn about the trials and tribulations of survivorship.

Alyssa Rieber is the chief of medical oncology at the Lyndon B. Johnson General Hospital. She is also a cancer survivor who had to battle Hodgkin's lymphoma while trying to attend medical school. Writing in the American Society of Clinical Oncology's *ASCO Connection* newsletter, she shared her challenges with survivorship:

I found that I experienced two main crisis points during my cancer journey. The first was at the time of diagnosis, the "personal earthquake." The second was more surprising to me. It was at the end of treatment. At a time when I thought I would be celebrating, I found that I was anxious about how to adjust back to a normal life. I had been in crisis mode for many months and didn't know how to live a life not focused on cancer.

I talk about this with many patients and their families when their curative therapy is complete and they transition to surveillance visits. I let patients know that this is normal and that they need to be patient with themselves. Many times they experience stress when loved ones expect them to "snap out of it" and go back to the life they lived before. I explain to patients that they are typically changed forever by their diagnosis and will not be exactly like they were before.[5]

DEFINING *SURVIVORSHIP*

What does it mean to be a cancer survivor? The term is somewhat ambiguous. Does it mean you have survived the cancer and treatment, or is it synonymous with cure? Lori encounters this issue often:

> I am often asked by patients some variation of the question, How will I know if I am cured? Some patients want to understand the method by which we determine if they are cured, while others ask me if there will always be surviving cancer cells circulating in their bloodstream. While these are great questions, there are regrettably very few answers. For many cancers, there truly are cures, while for others we simply have to wait and see what happens over time. It is hard to be comfortable with that uncertainty. For the vast majority of patients, cure is something we can truly know only in hindsight after we follow patients over an extended period of time.
>
> Survivorship is a process that starts following active therapy. It is more inclusive than *remission* or *cure*. Its focus is not only on freedom from cancer but also on all the good health habits that can improve your wellness over the balance of your life.

Some experts argue that survivorship begins the moment a patient is diagnosed and begins treatment, while others insist that one must be cancer free for five years post-treatment to earn this title. Perhaps by looking at the origins of the term and research conducted with patients regarding attitudes toward survivorship, we can agree on an appropriate definition.

The first use of the term *survivorship* is attributed to a physician, Fitzhugh Mullan, who had been diagnosed with cancer in the 1980s: "Mullan believed that the simple concept of cure did not capture the long-term experience of cancer and described survivorship as an independent phenomenon with unique challenges facing cancer survivors."[6]

Mullan's work helped to kindle a growing interest in this unique time in the lives of cancer patients. Many research studies were subsequently conducted with cancer survivors. In one study, participants were asked to use a word or short phrase to define what *survivorship* meant to them. Here is what they said:

> "Conquering" was the most frequently mentioned meaning of survivorship (n = 36). Participants who defined survivorship as conquer-

ing spoke of displaying a particular strength and being victorious against an enemy, almost in military terms. One participant, for example, said that "[A] positive attitude had [helped me] overcome an invasion in my body."

"A new outlook" (n = 30) was defined as an increased awareness of one's mortality and appreciation of the value of time as well as newly discovered values and activities. One participant said, "I had to take a better look at what life is about. It also taught me that you can't really know what's going to happen from day to day."

Twenty women defined survivorship as "helping others," which included an interest in and behaviors directed toward assisting others, particularly other cancer survivors, in their journey. As one participant put it, "I need to be available to whoever would need me." The theme "free of cancer" (n = 24) was defined as feeling disease-free and alive. One participant said, "It means that I had cancer, that I'm rid of it, and I no longer have cancer in my system."

For 21 participants, being a survivor meant that life was "beyond one's control." They often described their survivorship as being in the hands of God or a result of luck. For instance, one participant described it as "not my time to leave this earth," and another felt as if she had won a prize. For seven participants, survivorship meant being part of a larger group that had a similar experience, or a "sisterhood." Two participants said of surviving, "It's a mark of distinction. You're one of a very exclusive club."

Four participants did not consider themselves survivors. Three of them did not see themselves as survivors because they thought they had not yet completed a process, underscoring the defining moment. A third participant said "it was only luck," underscoring the "beyond one's control" meaning.[7]

Based on Mullan's original intent in coining the term, coupled with the research on patients' associations with the term *survivorship*, Lori and I agree with Eva Grunfeld and Craig Earle's definition of *survivorship*: "The period after completing primary and adjuvant cancer treatment until recurrence or death is now recognized as a unique phase in the cancer control continuum. The term 'survivorship' has been adopted to connote this phase."[8]

THE CHALLENGES THAT AWAIT SURVIVORS

Regardless of when one becomes a survivor, survivorship often brings a host of new challenges to patients weary from battling cancer: "These challenges may be physical, psychosocial, practical, spiritual, or informational and can begin during treatment and persist beyond treatment (long-term effects) or occur months or years after treatment ends (late effects)."[9]

Many patients are caught off guard by the transition into survivorship. Just as they were adjusting to a new identity as a cancer patient, suddenly they have to redefine themselves as a survivor—all the while coping with new or ongoing sequelae of treatment. This sentiment was captured in a study of women with advanced ovarian cancer: "Women looked back at their experience as being somewhat surreal and realized that their lives had changed completely. A few women referred to it as 'stepping through the looking glass,' an analogy from Lewis Carroll, and described a feeling of being on the outside looking in, as if this were happening to someone else."[10] It's a time when "issues related to diagnosis and treatment diminish in importance, and concerns related to long-term follow-up care, management of late effects, rehabilitation, and health promotion predominate."[11]

THE GOOD NEWS: SURVIVORSHIP STATISTICS SHOW IMPORTANT GAINS IN EXTENDING LIVES

Thanks to advances in screening, diagnosis, and treatment of cancer, far more patients are now surviving their diseases for extended periods of time. In fact, the majority of patients suffering from breast, prostate, and colorectal cancer can look forward to a lengthy period of survival if not cure.[12] Many cancers have been transformed from a death sentence into a chronic or even curable disease: "Almost 80% of children and 60% of adult cancer patients are expected to survive at least five years from diagnosis and many of them are, in fact, cured from cancer."[13] In absolute numbers, there are approximately 14 million Americans living today who have battled cancer.[14]

These changes are extremely evident when examining survival rates. The American Cancer Society states, "The 5-year relative survival rate for all cancers diagnosed between 2003 and 2009 is 68%, up from 49% in 1975–1977. The improvement in survival reflects both progress in diagnosing certain cancers at an earlier stage and improvements in treatment."[15] As a result, the ratio between newly diagnosed cases of cancer and survivors is tipping increasingly in favor of survivors. Within twenty years, the number of newly diagnosed cancer cases worldwide will have doubled to more than 20 million, while the total number of survivors (here defined as people who have experienced cancer) will triple to 75 million.[16]

This population of survivors fits a certain profile: "The majority of cancer survivors (64%) were diagnosed 5 or more years ago, and 15% were diagnosed 20 or more years ago. Nearly one-half (45%) of cancer survivors are aged 70 years or older, while only 5% are younger than 40 years."[17]

It is important to note that survivorship statistics vary dramatically based on the type of cancer, stage, and other disease characteristics discussed in chapter 1. An example is breast cancer, where tremendous gains have been made due to better diagnostic and treatment modalities:

> It is estimated that there are nearly 3 million women living in the United States with a history of invasive breast cancer, and an additional 226,870 women will be diagnosed in 2012. The overall 5-year relative survival rate for female breast cancer patients has improved from 75.1% between 1975 to 1977 to 90.0% for 2001 through 2007. This increase is due largely to improvements in treatment (i.e., chemotherapy and hormone therapy) and to earlier diagnosis resulting from the widespread use of mammography. The 5-year relative survival rate for women diagnosed with localized breast cancer is 98.6%.[18]

EMOTIONAL CHALLENGES FOR SURVIVORS

Patients are often ill prepared for the stress of surviving cancer. As one research study revealed: "The transition from patient to survivor is often experienced as stressful as contact with the cancer care team decreases in frequency and the perceived safety of the hospital system is left behind."[19]

Dana B. shared the emotional toll of entering survivorship: "I felt that this is when the grieving started. This is when you need to deal with the psychological piece. I was grieving my body parts that weren't there. I was trying to find my 'new normal.' That's when the fears started to pop up. How was I going to, down the line, deal with these fears that pop up about this cancer coming back?"[20] Fortunately, Dana discovered that working with a psychologist could be very helpful and added, "Being a faithful woman, without God, I don't know how you do it. There's a devotional called 'Jesus Calling' that every day when I open the book, it speaks to me directly."[21]

Survivor distress is a common and wholly understandable phenomenon. The most frequent cause of distress is fear of recurrence. As Dana put it, "There are times when something is going on with my body—my back hurts, for instance—things that a normal, everyday person would just brush off. But the cancer survivor begins to think, 'What if this is the cancer that is coming back?'"[22]

The frequency and depth of distress that survivors experience appears to be governed by a host of factors:

- Whether the patient was prone to anxiety or depression prior to developing cancer. Dana shared: "My entire life, I've been a worrier. One thing that this experience has taught me is that worry is not going to change the circumstances I'm in. If you are worried day after day about something bad happening to you, then you are wasting your days. There's been a little mental adjustment for me."[23]
- The patient's diagnosis and prognosis (based on staging and other factors): In one study of approximately 1,300 survivors, the "percentage of survivors who reported anxiety, depression and comorbid anxiety-depression [was] highest among lung cancer survivors."[24]
- The degree of support the patient receives in addressing his or her concerns.

In a *New York Times* article, author Bruce Feiler chronicles the journey from cancer patient to cancer survivor and the emotional roller coaster he endured:

When I first learned that I had aggressive bone cancer in my left leg in 2008, I did what many patients do: I immediately searched out the five-year survival figures. I then did the grim calculation of how old my children would be at that time and whether I would outlive my parents. Over a brutal year of chemo, surgery, and rehabilitation, I kept an indelible ticking clock in my head. Sometimes I wondered, "Why won't the clock speed up?" Other times, "Why won't it slow down?" And as I slogged through subsequent years of scans—first every three months, then every four, then every six—and experienced what survivors call "scanxiety," I imagined what the five-year benchmark would feel like. Like an actor practicing my Oscar acceptance speech, I even rehearsed exactly what I would do: break down in tears, give a party, buy plane tickets to Hawaii. And yet, as I approached the milestone in recent weeks, I began to feel more ambivalence. What happened? Or had I been wrong all along?[25]

In addition to anxiety and depression, both men and women can also struggle with body image and sexuality. Treatment can cause hormones to be disrupted temporarily or permanently. Men undergoing treatment for prostate cancer frequently experience sexual dysfunction. The condition could resolve with time but not always. Colorectal surgery could also result in sexual dysfunction, a side effect for which patients are often unprepared.

The physical changes that women undergo following breast cancer surgery, particularly mastectomy, can result in a profound sense of loss and change in their body image. Dana shared, "I think what no one can prepare you for is the psychological defeminization feelings that come with it. And because I was not a candidate for immediate reconstruction, that just added to the emotional piece of living as a different female than I was before."[26]

Research studies have demonstrated that "physical abnormalities and low hormone levels resulting from . . . cancer therapy contribute to lower self-esteem, depression, less desire for sexual activity and lower libido. This is particularly significant for younger women undergoing breast cancer therapy and for those recovering from gynecologic malignancies."[27]

PHYSICAL CHALLENGES FOR SURVIVORS

It is beyond the scope of this book to list all of the potentially persistent, physical side effects that can appear during survivorship. Suffice it to say that virtually every body system can be permanently adversely affected by radiation, surgery, and chemotherapy. The younger you are at the time of treatment, the longer survivorship will potentially last—and the longer the period of time over which latent side effects can develop. Doctors and patients, whether adult or child, often face a trade-off between the adverse consequences of potent interventions and the dangers posed by the cancer itself.

WHO IS MY DOCTOR NOW?

For most patients, cancer defines their lives as well as their doctors for an intense period of time. As they transition from active treatment into survivorship, it's not always clear to whom they should turn for medical care. Lori comments, "In my practice, I would estimate that well over 50 percent of my patients ask me whom they should call with regard to new symptoms or medical concerns. Unfortunately, there is no clear protocol for differentiating the roles of the cancer specialist versus the primary care doctor."

The issue is of sufficient concern to attract the attention of the venerable Institute of Medicine (IOM), which identified this phase as a "time when the future role of the various healthcare providers is often unclear. For patients, it can be a time of confusion both about what follow-up care involves and about which physician is responsible for follow-up care."[28]

The IOM recommends, "Patients completing primary treatment should be provided with a comprehensive care summary and follow-up plan that is clearly and effectively explained." The report terms this the "Survivorship Care Plan."[29] A "Survivorship Care Plan" is intended to be a guide to help primary care physicians understand the nature of their patients' disease and treatment as well as the recommended follow-up regimen. Such plans should also include information regarding residual side effects or other medical issues resulting from cancer and its treatment that could require medical management.

Though it sounds simple enough, according to researchers Cowens-Alvarado and colleagues, "There are many barriers to the widespread implementation and use of such tools. The best evidence is that fewer than 15% of patients receive such a plan and that fewer than one-half of the National Cancer Institute-designated cancer centers consistently deliver care plans to their cancer survivors."[30]

Part of the problem is due to an imprecise definition of the respective roles played by cancer specialists and primary care physicians. A 2013 article by Klabunde et al., in *Family Medicine* brings this point home:

> We found that a majority of PCPs [primary care providers] perceive themselves as having an active role in the cancer-related follow-up care of survivors, most often in a co-management capacity with an oncologist. In contrast, most oncologists perceive that they directly provide cancer-related follow-up care themselves without much involvement from PCPs or other providers, a finding that parallels recent work documenting medical oncologists' limited engagement in co-managing breast cancer care.[31]

This is not an isolated finding, as revealed by the following research:

- "A majority (59%) of PCPs but only 23% of oncologists strongly or somewhat agreed that PCPs have the necessary skills to provide follow-up care related to the effects of breast cancer or its treatment. Similarly, 75% of PCPs, but only 38% of oncologists, agreed that PCPs have the skills necessary to initiate appropriate screening or diagnostic work-up to detect recurrent breast cancer. Only 8% of oncologists but 51% of PCPs believed that PCPs are better able than oncologists to provide psychosocial support for breast cancer survivors."[32]
- Potosky et al. state, "Our study also suggests that many PCPs—and even some oncologists—may lack critical knowledge or training to care for cancer survivors."[33] The study found that both PCPs and oncologists deviate from guidelines in caring for cancer survivors—though PCPs deviate more.
- "There is a growing consensus that inadequate follow-up care may be related to a fragmented health system that impedes communication and care coordination. Greater coordination of care be-

tween PCPs and oncologists has been shown to improve both the quality of and survivors' satisfaction with follow-up care."[34]

- "Many PCPs reported uncertainty about their own skill levels and lack of confidence in their knowledge of cancer survivor care. For example, less than 60% agreed that PCPs had the necessary skills to care for treatment effects in survivors of breast or colon cancer."[35]

It's understandable why patients would be confused!

Due to our highly fragmented health care system, communication breakdowns occur regularly during crucial hand-offs between physicians, such as during the transition to survivorship. While work is being done to standardize survivors' ongoing care, it's important that you work with your oncology team and primary care physician to agree on a survivorship plan that will meet your medical and wellness needs.

If you are interested in learning more about the IOM's research into the needs of cancer survivors, consider reading *From Cancer Patient to Cancer Survivor: Lost in Transition*.

In 2006, the Institutes of Medicine . . . published *From Cancer Patient to Cancer Survivor: Lost in Transition*, which focused on the specific needs of adult cancer survivors as they transition from cancer treatment to the post-treatment survivorship phase. This report was followed by a second IOM report, *Cancer Care for the Whole Patient: Meeting Psychosocial Health Needs*, which further emphasized the importance of assessing and treating the psychological, social, and spiritual issues experienced by many cancer survivors. Both reports recommended that survivors receive a detailed care plan to assess and treat the potential long-term and late effects specific to their cancer diagnosis and treatment. In addition, these reports emphasized the need to develop clinical guidelines for survivorship care and recognized the importance of primary care providers . . . as partners in the care of cancer survivors.[36]

ADVANCEMENTS IN SURVIVORSHIP CARE

Life will get better for survivors, and many of the deficits that currently exist will be addressed. That's the promise of the National Cancer Survivorship Resource Center (The Survivorship Center), which was created in 2010 as a collaborative effort by the American Cancer Society and the George Washington University Cancer Institute. The center receives financial support from the Centers for Disease Control and Prevention,[37] and its initial work focuses on addressing the need for survivorship care plans:

> Currently, The Survivorship Center has drafted follow-up care guidelines for patients with colorectal and breast cancer. Work is also underway to develop follow-up care guidelines for survivors of head and neck and prostate cancer.
>
> In addition to the work of The Survivorship Center, both the National Comprehensive Cancer Network (NCCN) and the American Society of Clinical Oncology (ASCO) are working to develop survivorship guidelines that address common long-term and late effects experienced by many survivors.
>
> The NCCN survivorship guideline incorporates information related to wellness as well as common long-term and late effects such as anxiety, depression, cognitive function, fatigue, sleep disorders, chronic pain, and sexual function. ASCO guidelines will focus on providing guidance for the clinical management of survivors, with an emphasis on the management of long-term and late effects such as treatment-related neuropathy. The NCCN also publishes guidelines for the management of most cancers that include surveillance for recurrent disease.[38]

These published guidelines are extremely useful to oncologists when discussing ongoing cancer surveillance and health maintenance issues. They are evidence based and readily available to incorporate into established follow-up care. According to Lori, "As a cancer patient and an oncologist, I would encourage you to ask your physician if there are published survivorship guidelines for your type of cancer."

POSITIVE ASPECTS OF SURVIVORSHIP

Beyond the obvious benefit of survivorship, many patients talk about the ways in which their lives have been changed for the better as a result of their experience with cancer. In a survey of 109 breast cancer survivors, 97 percent identified a benefit from their ordeal, including a new appreciation for life:

> The "new appreciation of life" (n = 95) involved being aware of one's own mortality and that time is a precious commodity. As a result, many participants said they would spend time more carefully with their loved ones and do the activities that they enjoyed most. Twelve participants said they now knew that "little things" were unimportant or that "little things" were actually the most important. However, in both cases, the meaning was the same. One participant said, "The little things aren't as important as I once thought they were. When I get upset over things, I stop and tell myself, 'Hey, I'm alive.'" Another participant described it a different way. "Everything is important in my life; every little thing. Breast cancer makes you more aware of what life is about."
>
> Improved relationships (n = 63) were positive changes in relationships with family members, significant others, and friends. Many stated that they had become closer to and more appreciative of others, and had developed some new bonds with other survivors. One participant said, "It is one of the best things that has ever happened to me; [it] made family relationships better."
>
> Self-improvement (n = 45) meant a change for the better in the person, such as an increase in emotional control (i.e., calm, stronger), becoming more compassionate toward others, developing new skills, or obtaining a degree. . . .
>
> Finally, 13 participants mentioned that a benefit of their experience was "spiritual change" which involved renewed faith, deeper sense of spirituality, and connection with God. As one participant explained, "It has led me to God. I learned a lot about myself, my life, and letting go of all those problems I was dealing with and looking at them in a different way."[39]

17

DIFFICULT DECISIONS AT THE END OF THE JOURNEY

Darrell H. recounts the time when Patricia's journey neared its end:

About the middle of 2012, Patricia started talking about having a lot of joint pain. It was harder for her to drive the car, so we went to see a rheumatologist, who suggested she try methotrexate. It really helped with her symptoms. He mentioned, though, that one potential side effect was that it could cause leukemia.

Patricia went in for a routine lab check in December 2012, and her white cells were six hundred on her lab work. The doctor told her to stay inside to lower her risk of infection. We thought maybe the medication was lowering her count. In January, she had a bone marrow biopsy at Menorah Medical Center, and her counts were not up. She went off the methotrexate.

By March, they identified a bad chromosome marker for MDS [myelodysplastic syndrome, a serious blood disorder often considered to be a precursor to leukemia]. Patricia asked, "Could this be from the methotrexate?" The doctor said, "You've had so many treatments over the past twenty years that we have no idea what caused it."

I still thought that this was manageable. After all, it's a *pre*-leukemia. Then there was the day that we went in to see Dr. K., thinking that we were going to have a treatment for MDS. He told us that the last bone marrow showed 58 percent blasts. "You have full-blown leukemia."

I thought back in time to the "Rituxan moment"—when I realized Patricia's fate came down to a coin flip. I became aware that there was a part of me that kept thinking we were going to win these coin flips; somehow, it is going to work. I was in this place until the day he told us it had turned into leukemia.

He told us we had two choices: palliative care or to participate in a clinical trial for AML. Patricia thought about it. She hated the idea of being in the hospital, but the trial offered a 50 percent chance of having a remission. Secondly, she said, "I've gotten so much out of medical research. If I can give something back that helps in some way, I want to do that." So she agreed to the clinical trial.

I took her to the University of Kansas Hospital on April 10. The chemo "worked" in that her bone marrow was empty, but they would have to wait to see what grew back. Her white count stayed stuck at around two hundred or three hundred. She was in the hospital for fifty-six or fifty-seven days. I tried to go down twice a day to see her. It was a grind. It was incredibly tough on her. Every window looked out on gray concrete.

On the Monday and Tuesday of the week of her discharge, she was still spiking a fever. On Thursday, they said she could come home, which came as a bit of a jolt to me. I remember sending out an e-mail update saying, "Okay, the same conditions that last night required a twenty-four-hour trained medical staff now requires one tired theologian to care for my wife." I became a little shaky about it.

We had to do platelet transfusions every few days. Then, completely out the blue, her blood cells shot up to 6.1. For about six weeks, she felt good. She went driving around town, shopping, yet probably knowing it was not going to last. About six weeks later, her counts dropped back down.

Things moved fairly quickly from there. The doctor said, "We have one treatment we can try. In about 25 percent of patients, it produces a nondurable remission." Well, in one sense, every remission is nondurable, so Patricia tried one week of it. Her mouth got terribly sore, and she ended up in the hospital for another week. She said, "Okay, that's enough."[1]

Throughout your journey, you will be assessing options, carefully considering every major fork in the road. The most difficult divide, however, is reached when you realize that cure might be an elusive goal. This truth could be revealed at the time of first diagnosis or much further along in the journey.

If you have arrived at this point, you may never reach the distant mountains that were once your destination. Even so, your journey could continue for months, years, even decades, bringing you much joy in the process. Some patients may feel a kind of calm in giving up the fight for a cure. Others may not wish to concede the battle and instead choose to exhaust every possible option.

There is no one right path to pursue. However, it will be of the utmost importance to make informed decisions based on accurate information about your disease, prognosis, and personal values.

Most cancer patients indicate that it is not merely how long they live with cancer but also the quality of life that they experience that defines this final stage of cancer. In an e-mail to his friends and family, Darrell summed up this point quite beautifully:

> Today is our thirty-eighth wedding anniversary. This was a less conventional way to spend it, but it has been a good day. Although, obviously, we would have preferred that the doctor had told us that Patricia's condition was minor and easily cleared up, as we've compared notes on the drive home (we stopped at Holy Land Café and got falafel sandwiches as an anniversary and postclinic treat—and a square of baklava for Patricia!), we find that we both have a basic sense of peace and well-being. We started telling each other back in '05, during and after Patricia's transplant with her own stem cells, "It's going to be okay even if it's not okay." We continue to live in that confidence, with the corollary belief that every day is a gift, and we want to be grateful for each one and to live each day as fully as we can. We will take them one at a time rather than fretting too much about trying to count them out in advance. We continue to be thankful for your friendship, love, and support.
>
> Joy and peace,
> Darrell[2]

WHAT PATIENTS EXPERIENCE

Every patient's journey is different, so we cannot describe precisely what you may experience if your cancer advances. What we do know, however, is that the symptoms will be determined largely by the locations of disease within your body, the extent or size of the primary tumor and metastases, and the degree to which your body's normal function is impaired by the disease process. The primary symptom for an advanced prostate cancer, for instance, may be pain due to extensive bone metastases, whereas a colon cancer patient may experience symptoms based on failure of the liver.

Some symptoms can dramatically affect your quality of life (QoL) and thus need to be controlled, including:

- chronic or intractable pain;
- nausea and vomiting;
- mental confusion, depression, and other cognitive affective symptoms;
- generalized weakness;
- anorexia and weight loss; and
- fatigue.

PALLIATIVE CARE AND QUALITY OF LIFE

This is the time when palliative care becomes important. Palliative care seeks to improve the QoL of patients who have a serious or life-threatening disease, such as cancer. The goal of palliative care is to prevent or treat as early as possible the symptoms and side effects of the disease and its treatment, in addition to the related psychological, social, and spiritual problems. The goal is not to cure. Palliative care is also referred to as comfort care, supportive care, and symptom management. A palliative care specialist is a health professional who specializes in treating the symptoms, side effects, and emotional problems experienced by patients.

Palliative care can help to find the balancing point between living an optimal amount of time with a difficult diagnosis and enjoying a quality of life that makes one's time meaningful. Palliative care can involve a team of providers:

Often, palliative care specialists work as part of a multidisciplinary team to coordinate care. This palliative care team may consist of doctors, nurses, registered dieticians, pharmacists, and social workers. Many teams include psychologists or a hospital chaplain as well. Palliative care specialists may also make recommendations to primary care physicians about the management of pain and other symptoms. People do not give up their primary care physician to receive palliative care.[3]

Because pain is one of the greatest factors affecting QoL for some cancer patients, it is a major focus for palliative care. For most cancer patients, pain is controllable. Allow me to repeat this statement because it is important for you and your caregiver to understand: The vast majority of cancer pain can be managed.

Your physician is trained to manage cancer pain and may do an excellent job of it. However, in a survey of six hundred oncologists published in 2012, researchers found significant variations in the quality of pain management.[4] It may therefore be beneficial to consult with a subspecialist whose sole focus is on addressing the needs of chronically ill patients, beginning with their pain. Palliative care specialists manage such needs.

WHEN IS PALLIATIVE CARE APPROPRIATE IN CANCER TREATMENT?

Palliative care can be given at any point during a patient's treatment when cure is not the primary goal. For some patients who are facing advanced disease at the time their cancer is discovered, palliative care ideally begins at diagnosis and continues throughout treatment.

A MORE IN-DEPTH LOOK AT PALLIATIVE CARE

According to the National Cancer Institute (NCI), palliative care can effectively "address a broad range of issues, integrating an individual's specific needs into care. The physical and emotional effects of cancer and its treatment may be very different from person to person. For example, differences in age, cultural background, or support systems may result in very different palliative care needs."[5]

The NCI defines four primary domains that could require attention as part of the palliative care process:

- **Physical.** Common physical symptoms include pain, fatigue, loss of appetite, nausea, vomiting, shortness of breath, and insomnia. Many of these can be relieved with medicines or by using other methods, such as nutrition therapy, physical therapy, or deep breathing techniques. Also, chemotherapy, radiation therapy, or surgery may be used to shrink tumors that are causing pain and other problems.
- **Emotional and coping.** Palliative care specialists can provide resources to help patients and families deal with the emotions that come with a cancer diagnosis and cancer treatment. Depression, anxiety, and fear are only a few of the concerns that can be addressed through palliative care. Experts may provide counseling, recommend support groups, hold family meetings, or make referrals to mental health professionals.
- **Practical.** Cancer patients may have financial and legal worries, insurance questions, concerns about their employment or about completing advance directives. For many patients and families, the technical language and specific details of laws and forms are difficult to understand. To ease the burden, the palliative care team may assist in coordinating the appropriate services. For example, the team may direct patients and families to resources that can help with financial counseling, understanding medical forms or legal advice, or identifying local and national resources, such as transportation or housing agencies.
- **Spiritual.** With a cancer diagnosis, patients and families often look more deeply for meaning in their lives. Some find the disease brings them more faith, whereas others question their faith as they struggle to understand why cancer happened to them. An expert in palliative care can help people explore their beliefs and values so they can find a sense of peace or reach a point of acceptance that is appropriate for their situation.[6]

THE BENEFITS OF PALLIATIVE CARE

When appropriate palliative care is integrated early into treatment, the benefits to the patient could be substantial:

Early palliative care intervention improves satisfaction with care, quality of life, and symptom control. Palliative care has traditionally been offered to patients late in the course of the disease, typically after all therapeutic treatment options have been exhausted. However, recent research has suggested that offering palliative care services earlier in the course of the disease leads to meaningful improvements in patients' quality of life and, in some cases, extends survival.[7]

There is evidence to support the role of palliative care in extending life:

> A prospective randomized study performed at the Massachusetts General Hospital enrolled newly diagnosed patients with non-small cell lung cancer into 2 groups. An intervention group consisted of patients assigned to receive early, concurrent, palliative care integrated with standard oncologic care, whereas the control group received only standard oncologic care. The findings were dramatic. Patients who received early palliative care were shown to have a better quality of life and fewer depressive symptoms, were more likely to have their resuscitation preferences documented, had a longer median duration of hospice care at end of life, and, most impressively, had a median survival that was significantly longer than the patients who received standard oncologic care (11.6 vs. 8.9 months) in spite of receiving less disease-modifying and life-prolonging treatment.
>
> A previous retrospective study, which analyzed Medicare claims databases for selected cohorts of Medicare beneficiaries (n = 4493) for 5 types of cancer and congestive heart failure patients, found that mean survival was 29 days longer for patients enrolled in hospice than for non-hospice patients. In particular, the mean survival was significantly longer for hospice patients with congestive heart failure, lung cancer, pancreatic cancer, and marginally significantly longer for patients with colon cancer.[8]

The following is a brief summary of important facts about palliative care designed to eliminate misperceptions that patients commonly hold about this important service.

IS PALLIATIVE CARE ONLY FOR THE DYING?

There is a commonly held misperception that palliative care physicians only address the needs of the dying. Granted, palliative care physicians do care for hospice patients, but they do so much more. Palliative care simply means that your cancer has become a chronic (incurable) condition and the goals of treatment have shifted from being curative to slowing the progression of the disease while maximizing the quality of your life.

IF A PERSON ACCEPTS PALLIATIVE CARE, DOES IT MEAN HE OR SHE WON'T GET CANCER TREATMENT?

No. Palliative care can occur concurrently with cancer treatment, including chemotherapy or radiation. The focus of your oncologist remains treating the cancer, while the focus of the palliative care team is to work side by side with your oncologist to manage your symptoms. However, when a patient reaches a point at which active cancer treatment is no longer warranted, palliative care can become the primary focus of care. It will continue to be given to alleviate the symptoms and emotional issues of cancer. Palliative care providers can help ease the transition to end-of-life care.

A WELCOME HAND WHEN THE PATH NARROWS

You might think of a palliative care specialist as someone who gently lifts the backpack off your travel-weary shoulders and helps you through the remaining part of your journey. He or she understands not only pain, but also the myriad other issues that can make survivorship less of a blessing and more of a hardship for you as well as for your caregiver. Once again, it is helpful to refer to the NCI's information on the scope of services provided by palliative care as well as those eligible to receive it.

WHAT IS THE DIFFERENCE BETWEEN PALLIATIVE CARE AND HOSPICE?

Although hospice care has the same principles of comfort and support, palliative care begins earlier in the disease process. As noted earlier, a person's cancer treatment can continue to be administered and assessed while he or she is receiving palliative care.

Hospice care is a form of palliative care for patients whose therapies are no longer controlling the disease and for whom active treatment has stopped. It focuses on caring, not curing. When a person has a terminal diagnosis (usually defined as having a life expectancy of six months or less) and is approaching the end of life, he or she becomes an appropriate candidate for hospice care.

YOUR CAREGIVER'S REACTION TO PALLIATIVE CARE

Your caregivers will also struggle with this existential fork in the road. It is completely natural for them to feel torn between wanting what is best for you and not wanting to ever give up. Others may be worn out by the journey you have traversed together and be more accepting of fate:

> It's common for family members to become overwhelmed by the extra responsibilities placed upon them. Many find it difficult to care for a relative who is ill while trying to handle other obligations, such as work and caring for other family members. Other issues can add to the stress, including uncertainty about how to help their loved one with medical situations, inadequate social support, and emotions such as worry and fear. These challenges can compromise their own health. Palliative care can help families and friends cope with these issues and give them the support they need.[9]

The more openly and honestly you communicate with your caregivers, the more likely that this will be a time of great emotional healing for all.

YOUR DECISIONS SHOULD BE BASED ON A CLEAR UNDERSTANDING OF YOUR MEDICAL CONDITION

Patients often forgo palliative care in favor of staying focused on active and aggressive treatment. There is mounting evidence from studies suggesting that some such decisions may be due to patients' lack of understanding of the true status of their condition and the goals of treatment:

Most patients with these so-called stage 4 cancers who choose to undergo chemotherapy seem to believe, incorrectly, that the drugs could render them cancer-free. That is the finding of a recent national study of nearly 1,200 patients with advanced cancers of the lung or colon. Overall, 69 percent of those with stage 4 lung cancer and 81 percent of those with stage 4 colon cancer failed to understand "that chemotherapy was not at all likely to cure their cancer," Dr. Jane C. Weeks, an oncology researcher at the Dana-Farber Cancer Institute in Boston, and colleagues reported in *The New England Journal of Medicine*.[10]

It is important to note that the choices we make can have a profound impact on the time we have remaining in our journey:

In the SUPPORT study, cancer patients who were over 90% sure they would live for at least 6 months were over two and a half times more likely to favor life-extending therapy over symptom-focused care compared with those who thought there was even a 10% chance they would not live 6 months. Those preferring life-extending therapy were more likely to undergo aggressive therapy, but their 6-month survival was no better than the more pessimistic group. Instead, they were more likely to have a readmission to hospital, an attempted resuscitation, or a death whilst receiving ventilator assistance. Another American study found patients who were aware they are terminally ill were more likely to discuss end-of-life care with their physician and more likely to receive care that was consistent with their wishes.[11]

Would these same patients have undergone difficult therapies if they knew they were not curative, or might they have elected for a less difficult path with fewer side effects and greater QoL? The only way to answer these questions is by providing patients with the required information to make truly informed decisions.

A NOTE TO PHYSICIANS

As discussed in chapter 2, physicians are not always forthcoming about a patient's condition and prognosis. After all, it is not easy to share life-altering information. Sometimes a patient's future truly is uncertain, and physicians don't like to offer survival numbers that may take away hope. Hence, it is understandable why physicians would rather avoid initiating such difficult conversations. Not only are these discussions emotionally taxing, but also they require time—a commodity in increasingly short supply for most physicians.

Studies have explored levels of physician disclosure and come to the following conclusions:

> Patients with incurable disease state that they want truthful information about their diagnosis, treatment options, and course even if the outlook is poor; but most patients never receive information from their physicians about prognosis or even imminent death. . . .
>
> Despite nearly all American patients stating that they want full disclosure about their prognosis, treatment options, and expected outcomes, most patients do not receive such information or receive such information far too late in their course.[12]

No one wants to confront his or her own mortality, yet patients clearly desire empathic and honest disclosure by their physicians about their disease progression and prognosis. Lori adds, "For those unfortunate patients who do not have hope for long-term survival, it is essential for us, as physicians, to take time to communicate that to our patients and their caregivers in a compassionate and sensitive manner. Such communication will allow for honest, open dialogue that improves our ability to meet patients' end-of-life goals."

PHYSICIANS ARE CONCERNED OVER PATIENT REACTIONS TO A CONVERSATION ABOUT PALLIATIVE CARE

Some physicians also express concern that frank conversations about palliative care versus curative care could remove hope and cause the patient to spiral into depression. Accordingly, they shield patients from the reality of their conditions. Here's what the prestigious *Journal of Clinical Oncology* had to say about the myths commonly held by physicians regarding sharing a patient's palliative status:

It Will Make People Depressed. Incorrect. In fact, giving patients honest information may allow them and their caregivers to cope with illness better. In the Coping With Cancer study, patients who reported having end-of-life discussions had no higher rates of depression or worry and had lower rates of ventilation and resuscitation and more and earlier hospice enrollment. More aggressive medical care at the end of life was associated with a higher risk of major depressive disorder in bereaved caregivers.

These are associations, and it is possible that in a randomized trial of telling the truth to half and withholding it from others, some of the informed group would object. But such a trial would be unethical. Most people—90% in most recent surveys of patients with cancer—want to know their prognosis. Physicians who ask, "What do you know about your illness? What do you want to know?" allow patients to express their own wishes about the information they want.

It Will Take Away Hope. Incorrect. In fact, evidence suggests that hope is maintained even with truthful discussions that teach the patient that there is no chance of cure. In an advanced cancer population, patients who were given a poor prognosis, low likelihood of response to treatment, and no chance of cure remained hopeful about their futures. . . . Similarly, hope was increased or at least preserved when parents of pediatric patients were given prognostic information, even if the news was bad. It is striking that physician honesty, even about difficult news, may actually help patients to feel more hopeful. . . .

Involvement of Hospice or Palliative Care Will Reduce Survival. Incorrect. Multiple studies suggest that survival is equal or better with hospice or palliative care. Among 4,493 Medicare beneficiaries who died after a diagnosis of congestive heart failure or one of five cancers, hospice use was associated with increased survival. Patients with lung cancer who use hospice have a better chance of being alive at 1 and 2 years, and chemotherapy use during the last 2 weeks of life did not improve their survival but did delay hospice enrollment. [13]

If oncologists listened carefully to palliative patients, they would likely hear a very clear request by the patients to understand their prognosis so as to facilitate astute decisions going forward, as was revealed in these research findings from a study of 126 patients with metastatic cancer sourced from 30 oncologists and recently diagnosed (within 6–8 weeks of recruitment for participation in the study):

> Ninety-eight percent of patients wanted their doctor to be realistic, provide an opportunity to ask questions, and acknowledge them as an individual when discussing prognosis. Doctor behaviors rated the most hope giving included offering the most up to date treatment (90%), appearing to know all there is to know about the patient's cancer (87%), and saying that pain will be controlled (87%). The majority of patients indicated that the doctor appearing to be nervous or uncomfortable (91%), giving the prognosis to the family first (87%), or using euphemisms (82%) would not facilitate hope.[14]

IT'S NOT WHAT YOU SAY BUT HOW YOU SAY IT

Before concluding this chapter, we wish to share a final message to our physician partners on the journey. Patients will tell you that one thing can make a huge difference:

> How and how often doctors discuss options with patients and describe the potential of continued treatment. [It was] suggested that practitioners master "the conversation known as 'ask, tell, ask,' which consists of asking patients what they want to know about their prognosis, telling them what they want to know, and then asking, 'What do you now understand about your situation?'"[15]

18

CHOOSING TO STOP TREATMENT AND THE ROLE OF HOSPICE

Randy Pausch was a beloved professor of computer science at Carnegie Mellon University in Pittsburgh, Pennsylvania. In 2006, he was diagnosed with pancreatic cancer, a disease that would claim his life in 2008. Randy wrote a book about coping with his disease called *The Last Lecture*. An abridged version was posted online and received well over six million views. Here's a glimpse into his powerful story:

> I'm hanging in there, trying to spend as much quality time with my wife and kids as possible, and though it's very frustrating to know I won't beat the cancer, there's a great satisfaction in knowing that I'm walking off the field with no regrets.
>
> I am dying soon, and I am choosing to have fun today, tomorrow and every other day I have left.[1]

THE JOURNEY NEARS ITS END

For some patients, cancer will progress to a point where only supportive care is appropriate as they prepare to transition from life. They may be in the ICU of a major hospital when this time arises or at home being cared for by their family. Where and how the patient dies will be determined primarily by their preparation for this final stage of life.

Darrell H. recalled a conversation with their palliative care physician, who offered guidance about when one knew it was time to stop active treatment:

> We had been seeing Dr. W. in the palliative care department. He really was outstanding. One of the things he had said sometime earlier, in response to her question about when she would know to switch from palliative care to hospice, was that one of the signs might be when it was too much physical effort to get to the clinic. That was a guidepost for her. She thought, "You know, it would be kind of a relief not to have to run down to the clinic every few days and instead stay home." But certainly the miserable last week that she spent in the hospital helped her say, "I'm done. I don't want to do this anymore." Plus, there just weren't any good remaining options.
>
> Even so, as she proceeded from active treatment to palliative treatment en route to hospice, Patricia struggled with the notion of giving up. Our counselor said, "Here's the way I look at it. You are not giving up. You are shifting what you are fighting for. You are shifting from fighting for length of life to fighting for the quality of life you want. You are saying, 'This is the way I want to handle this process.'"[2]

THE ROLE OF HOSPICE

If you or someone you love has reached this point, hospice can be a tremendously valuable resource. Hospice is not a surrendering to death but rather respecting the importance of maintaining some semblance of quality of life while being surrounded by one's loved ones in the final stages of a disease. Hospice is for patients who have decided to forgo active treatment to prevent the further spread of their disease in favor of comfort care. Medicare covers hospice for patients deemed to be within six months of dying.

THE ORIGIN OF HOSPICE

Throughout this book, our metaphor has been that of a journey, so it is fitting to draw our book to a conclusion discussing a term associated with long journeys:

The term "hospice" (from the same linguistic root as "hospitality") can be traced back to medieval times when it referred to a place of shelter and rest for weary or ill travelers on a long journey. The name was first applied to specialized care for dying patients by physician Dame Cicely Saunders, who began her work with the terminally ill in 1948 and eventually went on to create the first modern hospice—St. Christopher's Hospice—in a residential suburb of London.[3]

Hospice care in America formally began forty years ago, when Florence Wald, dean of Yale's School of Nursing, joined forces with two physicians and a chaplain to found the inaugural hospice in Branford, Connecticut.[4] Wald's work was built on a foundation laid by several prominent physicians who were convinced that there was a better way for patients to transition from life than dying in the sterile confines of a hospital.

Among the most vocal of these physicians was Elisabeth Kübler-Ross. As a result of her publication of the landmark book *On Death and Dying*, Kübler-Ross had become recognized as the definitive expert on the dying process. In 1972, she was invited to testify before a Senate committee investigating the topic of dying with dignity. Here is an excerpt from that testimony:

> We live in a very particular death-denying society. We isolate both the dying and the old, and it serves a purpose. They are reminders of our own mortality. We should not institutionalize people. We can give families more help with home care and visiting nurses, giving the families and the patients the spiritual, emotional, and financial help in order to facilitate the final care at home.[5]

Despite a difficult start, hospices began to appear across the nation. Over time, the movement gained substantial momentum. Today, an estimated 5,500 programs provide hospice services to more than 1.5 million people annually.[6] This growth can be seen in a simple statistic from Medicare: "Of all Medicare decedents in the year 2001, 18.8% accessed hospice for three or more days. By 2007 the proportion of Medicare decedents accessing three or more days of hospice services had increased to 30.1%."[7]

SEEKING A NONMEDICALIZED DEATH

One of the goals of hospice is to provide a nonmedicalized death, a topic I discuss in *The Myths of Modern Medicine*:

> Rather than being driven by technology, the other path at the end of life is driven by the heart. It begins with an acceptance of the patient's condition and a desire to make this final stage of life meaningful. It requires a committed team of caregivers whose focus is on making the patient comfortable, pain free, and able to bring closure to their lives. In America, it is the path less traveled.[8]

This path leads to a very different experience for patients and caregivers: "If a patient is allowed to terminate his life in the familiar and beloved environment, it requires less adjustment for him. His own family knows him well enough to replace a sedative with a glass of his favorite wine, or the smell of a home-cooked soup may give him the appetite to sip a few spoons of fluid, which, I think is still more enjoyable than an infusion."[9] It is a gift not only to the patient but also to all who participate in the dying process.

For most people, that means removing the patient from the stark and sterile confines of a hospital so that he or she can spend remaining time surrounded by family at home.

RICK'S DECISION

The doctors at MD Anderson told Rick that he had reached a point in the journey where they had nothing more to offer him. His local oncologist, Dr. B., suggested that he try one more treatment. It didn't work either. Rick started to have seizures, requiring him to be on antiseizure medication. Diane recounts:

> We got to a point where Dr. B. advised that we could try and use CyberKnife [a focused form of radiation therapy] to reduce the size of the tumors, but it would not extend his life. She asked Rick what he wanted to do with the few months of life he had left. He was done.
>
> We started hospice at home, not knowing how much time we had. I took leave. Hospice gave us the opportunity for me to

be his wife and for our friends to come by and pay their respects.[10]

CARE NEEDS OF HOSPICE PATIENTS

Though people's needs vary greatly as death approaches, certain concerns are common among many patients. Patients may agonize over being a burden to their families or, conversely, of being abandoned. They may fear losing control and, with it, their dignity. Caregivers can help alleviate these burdens through some simple actions outlined by the National Cancer Institute:

- Keep the person company. Talk, watch movies, read, or just be with him or her.
- Allow the person to express fears and concerns about dying, such as leaving family and friends behind. Be prepared to listen.
- Be willing to reminisce about the person's life.
- Avoid withholding difficult information. Most patients prefer to be included in discussions about issues that concern them.
- Reassure the patient that you will honor advance directives, such as living wills.
- Ask if there is anything you can do.
- Respect the person's need for privacy.
- Support the person's spirituality. Let them talk about what has meaning for them, pray with them if they'd like, and arrange visits by spiritual leaders and church members, if appropriate. Keep objects that are meaningful to the person close at hand.[11]

Darrell and Patricia began their conversations about death early in their journey:

Clear back to 2001, when the first two treatments did not work, Patricia said, "You know, I really need to decide if I believe the things I say I believe. Jesus said, in John 14, 'I go to prepare a place for you. I'll be ready to receive you.' Do I really believe that?"

She took this very seriously. She thought about it. She prayed about it. She wrote about it. And then she said, "I'm at peace with dying. I do believe what I said I believe." And in this last year, she refined her thinking. She said, "I'm at peace with being dead, but the process of dying scares me. I don't know what kind of pain there is going to be." She felt as though all pain medications would make her sick to her stomach. The prospect scared her. Fortunately Zofran [an antinausea medicine] really helped her.[12]

THE ROLE OF FAMILY IN HOSPICE CARE

The National Hospice and Palliative Care Organization provides a valuable perspective on the role family members play in hospice care.

Typically, a family member serves as the primary caregiver and, when appropriate, helps make decisions for the terminally ill individual. Members of the hospice staff make regular visits to assess the patient and provide additional care or other services. Hospice staff is on-call 24 hours a day, seven days a week. The hospice team develops a care plan that meets each patient's individual needs for pain management and symptom control. The interdisciplinary team . . . usually consists of the patient's personal physician, hospice physician or medical director, nurses, hospice aides, social workers, bereavement counselors, clergy or other spiritual counselors, trained volunteers, and speech, physical, and occupational therapists, if needed.[13]

The hospice team provides a variety of important services. The team:

- Manages the patient's pain and symptoms
- Assists the patient with the emotional, psychosocial, and spiritual aspects of dying
- Provides needed drugs, medical supplies, and equipment
- Instructs the family on how to care for the patient
- Delivers special services like speech and physical therapy when needed
- Makes short-term inpatient care available when pain or symptoms become too difficult to treat at home, or the caregiver needs respite

- Provides bereavement care and counseling to surviving family and friends.[14]

Lori and I each had a parent who died at home while under hospice care as well as a parent who died in the hospital. The difference between these experiences was profound. Because of hospice, the remaining times with our respective mothers are memories we cherish. It also helped to relieve the weight of caring for a dying loved one. Lori adds, "Even though I had practiced oncology for many years, when each of my parents were diagnosed with terminal cancers, it was important for me to give myself permission to remove my 'clinical hat' and put on my 'daughter hat.' It was a huge gift to be able to trust the medical care of the hospice professionals and focus on the precious remaining time we had with our beloved parents." Although Lori and I had been long-time supporters of hospice, it was not until we directly experienced its gifts that we realized what a profound difference it can make in the final days of one's journey.

AN UNDER-UTILIZED SERVICE

Despite its growth and inherent benefits, hospice is still under-utilized in the United States, with many patients continuing to die in the hospital: "Across the United States, about 29 percent of patients with advanced cancer died in a hospital between 2003 and 2007. The highest rate of hospital deaths was in Manhattan (46.7%). These rates were about six times higher than the rate in Mason City, Iowa, where only 7 percent of cancer patients died in the hospital."[15]

Despite significant growth in hospice care over the past three decades, unfortunately, many patients never learn of hospice or learn too late in the course of dying to benefit. Of those patients enrolled in hospice, many will fail to realize the full benefits because their admission was shortly before death: "In 2012, more than 1 in 3 received care for seven days or less, and nearly 9 in 10 received care for fewer than 180 days."[16] A patient will get more from hospice care if he or she participates early enough for hospice workers to build relationships with the patient and family. In an article for the *New York Times*, Jane Brody writes, "When patients pursue chemotherapy under the false belief that they still have a chance for a cure, it often delays their transition to the comfort care of hospice. When patients spend only a few days or a week in hospice, caretakers don't have enough time to get to know them and their families and offer the physical, emotional, and practical benefits hospice can provide."[17]

The reasons for this phenomenon are complex, but one of them surely centers on physicians' reluctance to give up the battle against cancer. These well-intended physicians may be unwilling to concede that death is an inevitable progression of some patients' disease, and at some point, the most healing aspect of care is to comfort the patient and family and to allow a gentle passing.

MAKING YOUR END-OF-LIFE WISHES CLEAR

Whether you receive hospice care could have less to do with your dying wishes and more to do with your location. For decades, a team of researchers at Dartmouth have studied geographic variations in medicine, often arriving at startling and disappointing conclusions regarding unwarranted and unexplainable variations in health care. Just as acute care is rife with such variation, unfortunately so, too, is care for the dying:

> Whether Medicare patients with advanced cancer will die while receiving hospice care or in the hospital varies markedly depending on where they live and receive care, according to the Dartmouth Atlas Project's first-ever report on cancer care at the end of life. The researchers found no consistent pattern of care or evidence that treatment patterns follow patient preferences, even among the nation's leading academic medical centers.
>
> Rather, with one in three Medicare cancer patients spending their last days in hospitals and intensive care units, the report's findings demonstrate that many clinical teams aggressively treat patients with curative attempts they may not want, at the expense of improving the quality of their life in their last weeks and months.
>
> The researchers examined the records of 235,821 Medicare patients age 65 or older with aggressive or metastatic cancer who died between 2003 and 2007. In at least 50 academic medical centers, fewer than half of these patients received hospice services. In some hospitals, referral to hospice care occurred so close to the day of death that it was unlikely to have provided much assistance and comfort to patients.[18]

There are steps you can take to ensure that you receive hospice care if or when appropriate:

> Experts strongly encourage patients to complete advance directives, which are documents stating a person's wishes for care. They also designate who the patient chooses as the decision-maker for their care when they are unable to decide. It's important for people with cancer to have these decisions made before they become too sick to make them. However, if a person does become too sick before they have completed an advance directive, it's helpful for family caregivers to know what type of care their loved one would want to receive.[19]

Critical documents related to one's end-of-life wishes need to be readily accessible. While the original copies can remain safely ensconced in a safety deposit box or file, copies should accompany you wherever you are receiving treatment. However, do not expect that the act of providing these documents to providers will ensure that your wishes are honored. As many caregivers have learned, it can take a powerful advocate to ensure that the medical community respects your dying wishes. In fact, a *New York Times* article published in June 2014 stated, "Researchers at the University of California, Los Angeles, surveyed more than 800 seniors and found that advance directives were not available in the medical records of more than half of the subjects who said they had completed and given them to a health care provider."[20]

If your wishes include hospice care, there are some important things you must know.

HOSPICES VARY SIGNIFICANTLY FROM ONE ANOTHER

Darrell, like most of us, was unfamiliar with hospice:

> I thought there was this big organization called "hospice," only to discover that there are all these different hospices out there. I would say, Get yourself informed, and be prepared to shop. We interviewed two different organizations and found an amazing amount of difference between the two of them. The difference was night and day. We had a wonderful experience with Grace

Hospice. They became like part of the family. I'm struggling with a little separation anxiety now![21]

Naomi Naierman has devoted her life to improving care of the dying. In 1995, she founded the American Hospice Foundation. Ms. Naierman reaffirms what Darrell discovered when shopping for a hospice provider. In an interview conducted by Paula Span of the *New York Times* in June 2014, Ms. Naierman strongly recommended asking a great many questions—and being wary if the hospice provider was hesitant to respond.[22] Ms. Naierman recommended questioning the provider about how long they have been in business in addition to obtaining answers about the following concerns:

- "Response times. That's part of hospices' standardized surveys. They ask family members, after death, whether the staff was available on weekends and on evenings. It's one of many measures that aren't available to the public yet, but it's a fair question to ask: What can you tell me about your staff's response time should I need your services on the weekend or on evenings? How long will I have to wait in an urgent situation?"
- "There comes a time when you're actively dying, in your last hours of life, and that calls for continuous care, 24/7. You want to ask whether it's their practice to keep a nurse or another clinician in the home when a patient is actively dying. Does the family get support? Do they see the patient through death?"
- "You would hope that in the last hours of life, a hospice would maintain its presence, especially if you're in your own home. But as the *Washington Post* just reported—and it was very disturbing—some hospices choose not to provide continuous care. In some states, a large percentage don't, which basically means that when you're actively dying, they don't stick around."
- "Another important question: Do you have an inpatient facility, in case my symptoms become complicated? Most hospices don't have their own facilities, but they can rent or manage a unit in a hospital or beds dispersed throughout a hospital or in a nursing home. The point is to have the capacity to manage your symptoms when they're not manageable at home."[23]

You need to scrutinize your final provider of care with the same rigor that you scrutinized your first.

TOURING AN INPATIENT HOSPICE

Earlier, we met Susan Gubar, a professor emeritus of English at the University of Indiana who has courageously shared her cancer journey through a series of articles in the *New York Times*. Writing in a piece published on July 24, 2014, Gubar spoke of her dread of suffering "anxiety, dementia, but mostly in pain" as part of the dying process. In an effort to assuage her fears, she agreed to go on a tour of a hospice facility where a friend had died:

> On a fearfully cold day, we drove to a lodge on a wooded lot at the edge of a small town. By a blazing fireplace surrounded by comfortable chairs, about 10 of us amassed—six women dealing with gynecological cancer and some of our husbands. We were quiet because the family of a patient was using the adjacent kitchen.
>
> The place was quiet and beautifully lit. Many rooms had French doors wide enough to open, in better weather, and through which a bed could be slid onto a deck overlooking the woods. There were paintings on the walls and upholstered chairs that converted into beds for caregivers.
>
> From the moment of diagnosis, I knew that I did not want to end up in a hospital, and especially not in the I.C.U.—with its blinking and beeping machines, its fluorescent lights never turned off, its frantic rhythms of intubations and C.P.R.s and codes and respirators, its endotracheal and feeding tubes, its infections and psychoses. It shocked me to learn that this is what happens to one out of five Americans.[24]

Although the vast majority of hospice patients die peacefully at home, it can be comforting to know that there are inpatient facilities dedicated to a nonmedicalized death where the patient is surrounded by loved ones. Like Susan Gubar, perhaps you and your family members would find a visit to a hospice comforting.

TALKING WITH YOUR DOCTOR ABOUT DEATH

I previously discussed the reluctance of many physicians to talk openly with patients about the course of their disease despite the fact that patients want to be apprised of their condition and prognosis. Research studies consistently demonstrate that doctors frequently fail to share information about the course of a patient's disease or impending death.[25] What patients and physicians may fail to realize is that "Not having a discussion about imminent death is associated with worse quality of care, worse quality of life, worse caregiver quality of life, and over $1,000 more in medical care cost in the last week of life."[26] We've learned a great deal about patient needs at the final stage of life:

> Communication about end-of-life care and decision making during the final months of a person's life are very important. Research has shown that if a person who has advanced cancer discusses his or her options for care with a doctor early on, that person's level of stress decreases and their ability to cope with illness increases. Studies also show that patients prefer an open and honest conversation with their doctor about choices for end-of-life care early in the course of their disease, and are more satisfied when they have this talk.[27]

> Many people believe that hospice care is only appropriate in the last days or weeks of life. Yet Medicare states that it can be used as much as 6 months before death is anticipated. And those who have lost loved ones say that they wish they had called in hospice care sooner. Research has shown that patients and families who use hospice services report a higher quality of life than those who don't. Hospice care offers many helpful services, including medical care, counseling, and respite care. People usually qualify for hospice when their doctor signs a statement saying that patients with their type and stage of disease, on average, aren't likely to survive beyond 6 months.[28]

> Various studies have shown that cancer patients in hospice live weeks to months longer than comparable patients not in hospice care.[29]

AS DEATH APPROACHES

The National Cancer Institute describes the following indicators that death may be approaching:

> Withdrawal from friends and family:

- People often focus inward during the last weeks of life. This doesn't necessarily mean that patients are angry or depressed or that they don't love their caregivers. It could be caused by decreased oxygen to the brain, decreased blood flow, and/or mental preparation for dying.
- They may lose interest in things they used to enjoy, such as favorite TV shows, friends, or pets.
- Caregivers can let the patient know they are there for support. The person may be aware and able to hear, even if they are unable to respond. Experts advise that giving them permission to "let go" may be helpful. If they do feel like talking, they may want to reminisce about joys and sorrows, or tie up loose ends.

Sleep changes:

- People may have drowsiness, increased sleep, intermittent sleep, or confusion when they first wake up.
- Worries or concerns may keep patients up at night. Caregivers can ask them if they would like to sit in the room with them while they fall asleep.
- Patients may sleep more and more as time passes. Caregivers should continue to talk to them, even if they're unconscious, for the patient may still hear them.

Hard-to-control pain:

- It may become harder to control pain as the cancer gets worse. It's important to provide pain medication regularly. Caregivers should ask to see a palliative care doctor or a pain specialist for advice on the correct medicines and doses. It may be helpful to explore other pain control methods such as massage and relaxation techniques.

Increasing weakness:

- Weakness and fatigue will increase over time. The patient may have good days and bad days, so they may need more help with daily personal care and getting around.
- Caregivers can help patients save energy for the things that are most important to them.

Appetite changes:

- As the body naturally shuts down, the person with cancer will often need and want less food. The loss of appetite is caused by the body's need to conserve energy and its decreasing ability to use food and fluids properly.
- Patients should be allowed to choose whether and when to eat or drink. Caregivers can offer small amounts of the foods the patient enjoys. Since chewing takes energy, they may prefer milkshakes, ice cream, or pudding. If the patient doesn't have trouble with swallowing, offer sips of fluids and use a flexible straw if they can't sit up. If a person can no longer swallow, offer ice chips. Keep their lips moist with lip balm and their mouth clean with a soft, damp cloth.

Awareness:

- Near the end of life, people often have episodes of confusion or waking dreams. They may get confused about time, place, and the identity of loved ones. Caregivers can gently remind patients where they are and who is with them. They should be calm and reassuring. But if the patient is agitated, they should not attempt to restrain them. Let the health care providers know if significant agitation occurs, as there are treatments available to help control or reverse it.
- Sometimes patients report seeing or speaking with loved ones who have died. They may talk about going on a trip, seeing lights, butterflies, or other symbols of reality we can't see. As long as these things aren't disturbing to the patient, caregivers can ask them to say more. They can let them share their visions and dreams, not trying to talk them out of what they believe they see.

The dying process:

- There may be a loss of bladder or bowel control due to the muscles relaxing in the pelvis. Caregivers should continue to provide clean, dry bedding and gentle personal care. They can place disposable pads on the bed under the patient and remove them when soiled. Also, due to a slowing of kidney function and/or decreased fluid intake, there may be a decrease in the amount of urine. It may be dark and smell strong.
- Breathing patterns may become slower or faster, in cycles. The patient may not notice, but caregivers should let the doctor know

if they are worried about the changes. There may be rattling or gurgling sounds that are caused by saliva and fluids collecting in the throat and upper airways. Although this can be very disturbing for caregivers, at this stage the patient is generally not experiencing any distress. Breathing may be easier if a person's body is turned to the side and pillows are placed behind the back and beneath the head. Caregivers can also ask the health care team about using a humidifier or external source of oxygen to make it easier for the patient to breathe, if the patient is short of breath.

- Skin may become bluish in color and feel cool as blood flow slows down. This is not painful or uncomfortable for the patient. Caregivers should avoid warming the patient with electric blankets or heating pads, which can cause burns. However, they may keep the patient covered with a light blanket.[30]

WHAT HAPPENS AT DEATH

Sometimes talking about the process of dying makes it less scary. There are certain signs of an approaching death that can alert caregivers that the time of passing is near. Lori shares:

> When I have that very difficult conversation with patients and caregivers—explaining that their disease is no longer curable and it is time to refocus our efforts from treatment to comfort—I am inevitably asked what to expect at the end. A common refrain is, "How will I know?"
>
> I tell them that there are common signs that our physical body is preparing to leave this world, such as decreased appetite and sleeping more, but that every patient is different. I reassure them that most patients and their families have an inner sense about when death is approaching that they should trust. We as caregivers will walk beside them and help interpret these signs and help prepare them.

Darrell describes when he realized that death was close at hand:

> By early to mid-February, the hospice nurse said that she was seeing signs of Patricia's decline. She started getting low-grade fevers and had trouble swallowing. On February 16, I was taking Meghan on an outing. Dean and my two grandsons came over to spend a couple of

hours with Patricia. They were there when Meghan and I came by. It suddenly hit me that we had the whole family there, so I grabbed the camera, knowing that it might be the last time we had the whole family together. Looking back on it, she had nine days to live.[31]

A DEATH FULL OF GRACE

I want to share with you a gift that Darrell shared with the many people who cared so deeply for him and Patricia. In these final e-mails, Darrell allows us to walk along with him as Patricia takes the final steps of her long and courageous journey:

Hi, everyone—

First, the facts:

We've been told to expect this, and now we are starting to see some of the signs of decline in Patricia's physical condition:

1. She is having trouble swallowing—hospice has provided a thickening agent, and the thickened liquids go down more easily. We're cutting pills to swallow to a minimum.
2. She is more fatigued, although the level of that varies from day to day and partly depends on whether she has anything more interesting to do than talking to me.
3. She has more physical weakness—it's harder for her to get out of bed or walk around the apartment.
4. She has had more frequent low-grade (99° to 100°) fevers—about 3 mornings this week.
5. At times, though not very often, she is a bit more mentally fuzzy—not sure what day it is, or mixing up the order of events or the schedule.

Now, the feelings:

The list above sounds gloomy, a downer. But, somewhat to my surprise, the atmosphere around our house isn't really very gloomy. Oh, there are moments when I feel sad—if I see Patricia struggling with her morning coffee, choking and coughing, or if she has to work to recall a name or a place. And there have been moments this week when Patricia has felt sad, unsure of exactly what to expect as this all unfolds, or struggling with boredom as she lies in her bed. But, on the whole, she is still very much herself—she smiles and laughs easily.

We keep coming back, in our conversations, to the fact that Patricia is living with a sense of purpose, even though her strength and energy levels are greatly reduced. She wants to be a channel through whom God's love flows, to help and bless the people who are helping her in so many ways. And she is living with hope. She will say matter-of-factly, "I'm not going to be around here much longer. But I hope that, however things work on the other side of death, I can keep track of you and the kids and what's happening with the exciting projects at the church." She's collecting a list of names that people have asked her to look up and give a hug to in eternity—I'd never thought of that kind of a "to-do list" before.

Today she and I were sharing a couple of short paragraphs Phillip Yancey wrote in his book *The Jesus I Never Knew*. They go like this:

"There are two ways to look at human history, I have concluded. One way is to focus on the wars and violence, the squalor, the pain and tragedy and death. From such a point of view, Easter seems a fairy tale exception, a stunning contradiction in the name of God . . . . There is another way to look at the world. If I take Easter as the starting point, the one incontrovertible fact about how God treats those whom he loves, then human history becomes the contradiction and Easter a preview of ultimate reality. Hope then flows like lava beneath the crust of daily life."

Patricia listened, then softly repeated, "Hope then flows like lava." After a moment's thought, she said emphatically, "I *like* that!" And so do I.

Joy, peace—and hope,
Darrell[32]

On February 25, 2014, as Patricia lay dying, Darrell wrote these words about her imminent passing:

A great light in our lives is growing dim. (Thank you to so many of you who have expressed the ways Patricia has impacted your life for good. Mine, too.) This is a painful loss. Patricia and I do not, however, believe it is a tragedy—nor do we believe that her light is lost forever but rather that it is relocating to a realm where it can shine more brightly and colorfully than ever. I can't wait to see what that will be like.

Joy and peace,
Darrell[33]

THE SURVIVING CAREGIVER

When a caregiver survives but the patient does not, he or she faces a difficult adjustment. They have spent weeks, months, or years with much of their life being defined by the care they bestowed on their loved one. Then, one day, their duties are no longer required, their loved one has passed, and they are painfully alone.

Despite having had twenty years in which to prepare, Darrell was stunned by the finality of his wife's passing: "The stark reality of standing there watching someone whom you've been with for thirty-nine years stop breathing puts the issue in a whole different focus than when you're sitting in a seminary classroom. This takes some real grappling."[34]

In our interview, which I felt so privileged to conduct, Darrell provided me with an unvarnished look into this painful time in his life. It yields a difficult glimpse into the role of the surviving caregiver:

> There were two things that I felt right away: One was relief, which was followed immediately by this sort of obligatory sense of guilt. I no longer have to listen, twitch, and jump at every noise from the other room. But combined with this feeling is an emptiness, a missing sense of purpose. There is something ennobling about being focused on the well-being of someone else. Then all of sudden there is a sense that no one needs you anymore.
>
> For me, there is also this sense that, now that I'm emerging from this caregiving stage, everyone else is already in the middle of their lives. No one has been saving a space for me. So how do I fit in out here? I cannot just call up a friend and say, "Hey, can we get together for dinner" because they have their own stuff going on.
>
> My folks were missionaries in Brazil, so I spent the first twelve years of my life in Brazil before we returned to the states. Now I am a seventh grader, and I go to school and the cliques are already there, and I do not understand the language about things like going steady. I felt like there was a rule book and everyone had a copy but me. It is

like the merry-go-round is whirling, and I'd like to get on, but it's going too fast.

One of the things that was very important to me was a concept given to me by our counselor. I had these feelings of guilt every time I left Patricia to do something that was rewarding to me—whether it was work or participating in fantasy baseball. Our counselor said, "Illness puts you in a completely different world. There is the world of the ill and the world of the well. The world of the ill throws you into a world where you don't know what to depend on. So it's really important to have fixed points that keep you in touch with the world of the well." The term *fixed points* became an important concept to me.[35]

Depth of feelings and profound insight obviously run in Darrell's family, as can be seen in how Darrell's son Dean managed the loss. Darrell recounts a recent memory from a bereavement support group session that he and Dean were attending:

Dean was asked to talk about what he had gotten out of the group. Dean said, "You know, when I came here, I was very angry, very angry about my mom dying. Then I had a breakthrough. There was one week when you asked us to write a letter to God. In that week, I suddenly had this moment when I realized that my mom had left me a trust fund. It wasn't a trust fund with money in it. It was far more precious and valuable than that. It was a trust fund filled with love. I realized that Mom had loved me enough to last me all of my life and that her dying did not take that away from me."[36]

Though Diane differed from Darrell by virtue of being both a cancer survivor and a surviving caregiver, she nonetheless experienced a shared sense of loneliness coupled with difficulty reintegrating socially without her partner:

Our friends still try to keep in touch, but it is so different. When you are a widow, you don't go out with the couples any more. The women call you when the men are busy and invite you out to dinner. That's hard to get used to. The first time I went to dinner with couples, they didn't know where to put me. Everyone was sitting across from their partner. It was so awkward. They, too, are missing Rick. It was just very hard.

I am very lonely, but I'm lonely for Rick. I just have to figure out what my new normal is, and I'm not anxious to find it! I don't want to forget a thing about my old life. At the same time, I don't want to live in the past. I'll just have to figure it out.[37]

THE ETERNAL POWER OF HOPE

Every doctor learns of the five stages of death and dying identified by Kübler-Ross. In an interview at her home in 1997, I had the privilege to ask Elisabeth what she would add to her work on death and dying, and she responded,

> I would add a chapter on hope. At the beginning, when people are diagnosed with cancer, their hope is always for a cure or at least for the prolongation of life. When they go through the stages, if they reach acceptance, you can diagnose it from the outside by asking them what is their hope. It never has anything to do with a cure or the prolongation of life. It has to do with things like acceptance by God in his garden. The quality of hope changes depending upon what stage the patient is in.[38]

So we leave you on your journey with this belief: "Overall, hope is probably the single most important element in the lives of patients and family members struggling with a diagnosis of cancer."[39] The journey may be arduous, but finding hope, regardless of one's outcome, brings a profound sense of meaning and closure to your life with cancer.

A FINAL WORD FROM LORI

It has been said that life has a way of coming full circle. I have come to realize this at a very personal level. After twenty-five years of practicing radiation oncology, I became a cancer patient. My reaction, like that of so many of my patients, was visceral—an overwhelming sense of fear and dread.

Cancer had already touched my life profoundly. I served as a caregiver for both of my parents throughout their individual battles with colon and ovarian cancers. I know what it feels like to be the person who wants to care for, support, and fiercely protect my loved ones.

Now, it was my battle. Sharing the same emotional roller coaster with my patients has increased my compassion, sharpened my sensitivity, and forever changed me for the better. My neat and tidy world was turned upside down.

I now see, from the patients' perspective, how a diagnosis of cancer ushers us into an unfamiliar world where we feel as though decisions must be made at breakneck speed—while we are struggling to assimilate overwhelming amounts of information often framed in an unfamiliar language.

Many nights over the dinner table or during morning coffee, my husband John and I would share ideas on how to ease the burden for cancer patients and their families. John has always been a strong patient advocate with a particular passion for addressing the psychosocial and spiritual needs of patients. Together, we felt as though we understood the totality of patients' needs at a critical juncture in their lives, which compelled us to write this book.

I have learned that treating cancer and coping with cancer are very different concepts. Our heartfelt goal is to distill overwhelming information into a logical, orderly sequence of steps that allows you to feel more knowledgeable, more empowered, and ultimately more in control of your destiny.

This reference guide will help you fill in the gaps that are often inadequately addressed by our health care providers, ranging from which questions to ask your physicians to nutrition, survivorship, and countless other issues. The journey can be difficult, but it can also be positively transformative for the patient and his or her caregivers.

Thank you for allowing us to share in this life-changing event. We pray you find this guide to be a useful resource during your journey.

RESOURCES

Lori and I have done our best to provide you with information that will help make your journey through cancer more manageable. Vast resources are available to you at no cost via the Internet and other venues.

What follows is a compendium of resources that you may find beneficial, many of which are located on the National Comprehensive Cancer Network (NCCN) website. We have taken much of this material directly from major, trusted websites. Although far from comprehensive, this list will provide you with a good launching point for exploring credible resources. We are grateful to a number of organizations for their efforts to empower patients with information, including:

- American Cancer Society (ACS),
- BMJ Evidence Centre,
- Cochrane Collaboration,
- National Cancer Institute (NCI), and
- NCCN.

ADVOCACY AND SUPPORT GROUPS

The mission of patient advocacy groups is to help make the journey through cancer less burdensome for the patient and family: "These groups work to ensure cancer patients receive appropriate and timely care, education, and financial assistance, when needed."[1] You can find a detailed list of advocacy organizations on the NCCN website at http://www.nccn.org/patients/advocacy/default.aspx.

GENERAL CANCER INFORMATION AND SUPPORT

Alliance of Dedicated Cancer Centers (ADCC)

ADCC is a national alliance of eleven, premier cancer institutions that are geographically distributed across the nation. "The ADCC member cancer centers play a pivotal role in the National Cancer Program, which was enacted by Congress in 1971 to improve the detection, prevention, diagnosis, and treatment of cancer. Unlike other hospitals, we are *singularly* dedicated to deepening the understanding of the causes and cures for cancer; developing new treatments for cancer; and disseminating this knowledge to the provider community at large."[2] These NCI-designated Comprehensive Cancer Centers may serve as invaluable resources for patients with rare or difficult-to-treat cancers, or as a source of a second opinion.

American Association for Cancer Research (AACR)

Founded in 1907 with the goal of furthering research into the causes of and cures for cancer, the AACR has grown into one of the most prestigious scientific organizations addressing the challenges of cancer.[3] In addition to publishing numerous peer-reviewed journals for physicians and researchers, AACR also publishes *Cancer Today*, the "authoritative resource for cancer patients, survivors, and caregivers who are seeking information and inspiration as they or their loved ones face diagnosis, treatment, and life after cancer."[4]

A wealth of consumer-directed cancer resources can be found on the AACR website at http://www.aacr.org/ADVOCACYPOLICY/SURVIVORPATIENTADVOCACY/PAGES/CANCER-RESOURCES-LISTING.ASPX#.VMuZ4kfF9oM. The organization can also be reached by telephone at (215) 440-9300, or toll free at 1-866-423-3965.

American Cancer Society (ACS)

The American Cancer Society provides a broad array of educational material on cancer and thus represents an excellent starting point for many patients and their families in the quest to learn more about the disease. ACS publishes detailed informational guides on topics ranging from the duties of a caregiver to pain management. In addition to their extensive online resources, ACS sponsors affiliated chapters in most major American cities.

The ACS website can be accessed at http://www.cancer.org/index. The toll-free telephone number is 1-800-ACS-2345.

American Society of Clinical Oncology (ASCO)

ASCO is a professional medical society founded in 1964 that represents more than 35,000 physicians and researchers from 120 countries who are involved in the study and treatment of cancer.[5] It is among the most highly regarded institutions dedicated to advancing the knowledge of cancer professionals. As part of its mission, ASCO produces a number of publications, including *The Journal of Clinical Oncology*. Telephone: (571) 483-1780; or toll free: 1-888-651-3038. ASCO also sponsors a consumer-directed site that can be accessed at www.cancer.net.

Association of Cancer Online Resources (ACOR)

ACOR offers information and support through its integrated system of online discussion groups. To further its mission, ACOR creates specific websites and also hosts a growing number of websites, created by:

- Patients for patients and caregivers. Many of those websites are considered to be clearly among the best sites for a particular disease or condition.
- Cancer Advocacy Organizations, many of which were created directly from the membership of an ACOR mailing list.
- Professional Organizations.

ACOR volunteers have also created a growing number of disease-specific websites.[6]

The organization can be reached via telephone: (212) 226-5525. Its website can be found at http://www.acor.org/.

Association of Community Cancer Centers (ACCC)

ACCC was founded more than forty years ago by community physicians dedicated to staying abreast of the latest research and treatment modalities and ensuring the highest standards for care delivered in a community setting. "Approximately 20,000 cancer care professionals from 1,900 hospitals and practices nationwide are members of ACCC. It is estimated that 60 percent of the nation's cancer patients are treated by a member of ACCC."[7] Most of the organization's resources are targeted toward oncology professionals. The website can be found at http://www.accc-cancer.org/. Telephone: (301) 984-9496.

Association of Oncology Social Work (AOSW)

> The Association of Oncology Social Work (AOSW) is a non-profit international organization dedicated to the enhancement of psychosocial services to people with cancer, their families and caregivers. Created in 1984 by social workers interested in oncology, AOSW has become the world's largest professional organization entirely dedicated to the psychosocial care of people affected by cancer.
>
> AOSW membership is comprised of an international set of professionals and students who practice in hospitals, cancer centers, home care agencies, hospice, community-based oncology practices, community programs, patient advocacy organizations, educational institutions and other settings.[8]

Numerous consumer-directed links to resources may be found at the AOSW website: http://www.aosw.org/aosw/Main/people-affected-by-cancer/resources-and-links/AOSWMain/People-Affected-by-Cancer/resources-and-links.aspx?hkey=ef31393a-d6ba-454d-87b2-bfeb9417fead. Telephone: (215) 599-6093.

Authentic Happiness

Authentic Happiness is a website sponsored by the University of Pennsylvania that provides detailed information about the field of positive psychology. One of the most useful aspects of the site is the numerous psychological tests you can take for free. These tests can help you determine the level of distress you are experiencing and whether some type of intervention may be helpful. Online: www.authentichappiness.sas.upenn.edu/.

Bone and Cancer Foundation

The Bone and Cancer Foundation provides a wealth of information for patients (and their families) who are suffering from bone-related cancer. The organization's tripartite mission is to:

- Provide information for cancer patients and family members on the causes and treatment of cancer involving bone.
- Provide information for physicians, nurses and other health professionals on the treatment of cancer involving bone.
- Advocate for increased government and private sector funding for research on cancer that involves the bone and related research areas.[9]

Its publication may be accessed via the web at: http://www.boneandcancerfoundation.org/. For more information, you may also call toll free: 1-888-862-0999.

CancerCare

CancerCare is among the top resources that cancer patients turn to for support:

> Founded in 1944, CancerCare is the leading national organization providing free, professional support services and information to help people manage the emotional, practical and financial challenges of cancer. Our comprehensive services include counseling and support groups over the phone, online and in-person, educational workshops, publications and financial and co-payment assistance. All Cancer-

Care services are provided by oncology social workers and world-leading cancer experts.

CancerCare programs and services help 170,000 people each year. We distribute 800,000 publications and welcome 1.5 million website visits annually. In the past year, CancerCare provided more than $22.3 million in financial assistance. The size and scope of CancerCare has grown tremendously since 1944, but it has never wavered from its mission of providing help and hope to people affected by cancer.

To learn more, visit www.cancercare.org or call 800-813-HOPE (4673).[10]

Cancer Experience Registry

"The Cancer Experience Registry is a community of people touched by cancer. The primary focus is on collecting, analyzing, and sharing information about the cancer experience, including the social and emotional needs of the patient and their family throughout the cancer journey."[11] A number of useful resources may be found on its website, including links to the Cancer Support Community: csc.cancerexperienceregistry. org/.

Cancer Hope Network

Cancer Hope Network is a national non-profit organization that provides free and confidential one-on-one emotional support to cancer patients, their caregivers, and their family members. Cancer Hope Network matches cancer patients or family members with trained volunteer cancer survivors who themselves, have undergone and recovered from a similar cancer experience.[12]

Toll free: 1-800-552-4366.

Cancer.net

Cancer.net provides timely, comprehensive, oncologist-approved information from the American Society of Clinical Oncology (ASCO), with support from the Conquer Cancer Foundation. Cancer.net brings the expertise and resources of ASCO to people living with cancer and those who care for and about them to help patients and their families make informed health care decisions.[13]

This site offers one of the most robust repositories of trusted information available, covering more than 120 types of cancer as well as related topics. It also provides essential tools that can help you find a cancer specialist and participate in support organizations, among other things. Online: http://www.cancer.net/. English and Spanish Patient Helpline: (571) 483-1780; or toll free: 1-888-651-3038. For printed materials: (703) 519-1430; or toll free: 1-888-273-3508.

The Cancer Project

Sponsored by The Physicians Committee for Responsible Medicine, The Cancer Project provides important information on nutrition, diet, and other topics that are significant to the cancer patient.[14] Its website is available at: http://pcrm.org/health/cancer-resources. Telephone: (202) 686-2210.

Cancer Support Community (CSC)

The Cancer Support Community is an international non-profit dedicated to providing support, education and hope to people affected by cancer. Likely the largest employer of psychosocial oncology mental health professionals in the United States, CSC offers a menu of personalized services and education for all people affected by cancer. Its global network brings the highest quality cancer support to the millions of people touched by cancer. These support services are available through a network of professionally-led community-based centers, hospitals, community oncology practices and online, so that no one has to face cancer alone. . . .

In July 2009, The Wellness Community and Gilda's Club Worldwide joined forces to become the Cancer Support Community. By helping to complete the cancer care plan, CSC optimizes patient care by providing essential, but often overlooked, services including support groups, counseling, education and healthy lifestyle programs. Today, CSC provides the highest quality emotional and social support through a network of more than 50 local affiliates, 100 satellite locations and online. See more at: http://www.

cancersupportcommunity.org/MainMenu/About-CSC/Who-We-Are. html#sthash.llOWFzcj.dpuf .[15]

Toll free: 1-888-793-9355.

Cancersymptoms.org

CancerSymptoms.org is dedicated to helping you find out more information about various symptoms you may have that could lead to early detection of various types of cancer such as liver, throat and kidney cancer. The website also features a number of resources to help you detect cancer earlier, as well as tips to help you cultivate a lifestyle that could prevent cancer altogether.

Read more: http://cancersymptoms.org/#ixzz3QJt4jGIE.[16]

Cancer Updates, Research & Education (CURE)

CURE magazine, launched in 2002 for cancer patients, survivors and caregivers, has become the largest consumer magazine in the United States focused entirely on cancer. With a circulation of 300,000, individual subscribers account for over 170,000 of that figure with the remainder going to cancer centers and advocacy groups around the country. Since its inception, CURE has expanded to reflect the entire cancer continuum, including supportive care issues and long-term and late effects.[17]

Telephone: (214) 367-3500; or toll free: 1-800-210-CURE.

LIVESTRONG

LIVESTRONG Foundation is one of the nation's leading cancer advocacy foundations, providing an array of tools for patients and their families, funding major research initiatives, and collaborating with like-minded organizations across the world. Since its founding, the organization has raised approximately $600 million to aid in the effort to conquer cancer.[18] Toll free: 1-855-220-7777. Online: www.livestrong.org.

National Cancer Institute (NCI)

The National Cancer Institute coordinates the National Cancer Program, which conducts and supports research, training, health information dissemination, and other programs with respect to the cause, diagnosis, prevention, and treatment of cancer, rehabilitation from cancer, and the continuing care of cancer patients and the families of cancer patients. Specifically, the Institute:

- Supports and coordinates research projects conducted by universities, hospitals, research foundations, and businesses throughout this country and abroad through research grants and cooperative agreements.
- Conducts research in its own laboratories and clinics.
- Supports education and training in fundamental sciences and clinical disciplines for participation in basic and clinical research programs and treatment programs relating to cancer through career awards, training grants, and fellowships.
- Supports research projects in cancer control.
- Supports a national network of cancer centers.
- Collaborates with voluntary organizations and other national and foreign institutions engaged in cancer research and training activities.
- Encourages and coordinates cancer research by industrial concerns where such concerns evidence a particular capability for programmatic research.
- Collects and disseminates information on cancer.
- Supports construction of laboratories, clinics, and related facilities necessary for cancer research through the award of construction grants.[19]

NCI is among the most important sources of information available to consumers, physicians, and researchers. Its website can be accessed at: http://www.cancer.gov/. Toll free: 1-800-4-CANCER.

National Center for Complementary and Alternative Medicine (NCCAM)

The National Center for Complementary and Integrative Health (NCCIH) is the Federal Government's lead agency for scientific research on complementary and integrative health approaches. We are 1 of the 27 institutes and centers that make up the National Institutes of Health (NIH) within the U.S. Department of Health and Human Services. The mission of NCCIH is to define, through rigorous scientific investigation, the usefulness and safety of complementary and integrative health interventions and their roles in improving health and health care.[20]

The website contains important information for any patient considering complementary and integrative modalities as part of their cancer treatment, including comprehensive information on herbal remedies. Visit its website at https://nccih.nih.gov/.

Toll free: 1-888-644-6226.

National Coalition for Cancer Survivorship (NCCS)

NCCS has worked with legislators and policy makers to represent cancer patients and survivors in efforts to improve their quality of care and quality of life after diagnosis. Our unique niche in the cancer advocacy landscape is promoting policy change to ensure quality cancer care. Our vision is to be an advocacy organization that reflects the needs of all cancer survivors to effect policy change at the national level.[21]

NCCS offers a number of valuable resources for cancer survivors and their families, which are available on its website at: http://www.canceradvocacy.org/. Toll free: 1-877-NCCS-YES.

The National Comprehensive Cancer Network

The National Comprehensive Cancer Network (NCCN), a not-for-profit alliance of 25 of the world's leading cancer centers devoted to patient care, research, and education, is dedicated to improving the quality, effectiveness, and efficiency of cancer care so that patients can live better lives. Through the leadership and expertise of clinical professionals at NCCN Member Institutions, NCCN develops resources that present valuable information to the numerous stakeholders in the health care delivery system. As the arbiter of high-quality cancer care, NCCN promotes the importance of continuous quality improvement and recognizes the significance of creating clinical practice guidelines appropriate for use by patients, clinicians, and other health care decision-makers.[22]

As part of its mission, the NCCN distributes treatment guidelines for specific disease conditions. This information often exists in one of two forms—the first intended for use by physicians, and the other aimed at consumers. NCCN can be accessed at: http://www.nccn.org.

National Hospice and Palliative Care Organization (NHPCO)

The National Hospice and Palliative Care Organization (NHPCO) is the largest nonprofit membership organization representing hospice and palliative care programs and professionals in the United States. The organization is committed to improving end of life care and expanding access to hospice care with the goal of profoundly enhancing quality of life for people dying in America and their loved ones.[23]

English and Spanish Helpline: 1-800-658-8898.

National Organization for Rare Diseases (NORD)

NORD offers a phenomenal compendium of information on rare diseases and genetic conditions:

The National Organization for Rare Disorders (NORD), a 501(c)(3) organization, is a unique federation of voluntary health organizations dedicated to helping people with rare "orphan" diseases and assisting the organizations that serve them. NORD is committed to the identification, treatment, and cure of rare disorders through programs of education, advocacy, research, and service.[24]

Online: http://www.rarediseases.org/. Toll free: 1-800-999-NORD.

Oncology Nursing Society (ONS)

The Oncology Nursing Society (ONS) is a professional association of more than 35,000 members committed to promoting excellence in oncology nursing and the transformation of cancer care. Since 1975,

ONS has provided a professional community for oncology nurses, developed evidence-based education programs and treatment information, and advocated for patient care, all in an effort to improve quality of life and outcomes for patients with cancer and their families. Together, ONS and the cancer community seek to reduce the risks, incidence, and burden of cancer by encouraging healthy lifestyles, promoting early detection, and improving the management of cancer symptoms and side effects throughout the disease trajectory.[25]

The organization's primary focus is on the oncology nursing professional. http://www.ons.org. Telephone: (412) 859-6100; or toll free: 1-866-257-4667.

Patient Advocate Foundation

Patient Advocate Foundation (PAF) is a national 501(c)(3) non-profit organization which provides professional case management services to Americans with chronic, life threatening and debilitating illnesses. PAF case managers serve as active liaisons between the patient and their insurer, employer and/or creditors to resolve insurance, job retention and/or debt crisis matters as they relate to their diagnosis. . . . Patient Advocate Foundation seeks to safeguard patients through effective mediation assuring access to care, maintenance of employment and preservation of their financial stability.[26]

Online: http://www.patientadvocate.org/. Toll free: 1-800-532-5274.

Prevent Cancer Foundation

Since 1985, the Prevent Cancer Foundation, a 501(c)(3) nonprofit, has invested $138 million in support of cancer prevention research, education, advocacy and outreach programs nationwide and has played a pivotal role in developing a body of knowledge that is the basis for important prevention and early detection strategies. The Foundation is the only U.S. nonprofit organization solely devoted to cancer prevention and early detection. We have funded nearly 450 scientists at over 150 leading medical institutions across the country. Our public education programs have applied this scientific knowledge to inform the public about ways they can reduce their cancer risks. See more at: http://www.preventcancer.org/what-we-do/#sthash.8zLJfQR3.dpuf.[27]

Toll free: 1-800-227-2732.

RESOURCES FOR INFORMATION ON CLINICAL TRIALS

The roster of clinical trials changes on a daily basis, with new trials being added and others being closed to enrollment. You should begin your search by speaking with your physician, who will be in the best position to assess your eligibility to participate in certain trials. If you wish to explore clinical trials on your own, there are a number of organizations that provide listings, including the following resources.

Center for Information and Study on Clinical Research Participation (CISCRP)

CISCRP allows patients to search for various clinical trials at https://www.ciscrp.org/programs-events/search-clinical-trials/. Toll free: 1-877-MED-HERO.

CenterWatch

CenterWatch is the oldest source of web-based, comprehensive information on clinical trials. Its website states:

> Founded in 1994, CenterWatch is a trusted source and global destination for clinical trials information for both professionals and patients. Located in Boston, CenterWatch provides proprietary data and information analysis on clinical trials through a variety of newsletters, books, databases, and information services used by pharmaceutical and biotechnology companies, CROs, SMOs, and investigative sites involved in the management and conduct of clinical trials.[28]

It should be noted that it is *not* a not-for-profit organization or foundation, and its information should not be construed as an endorsement for the validity of any particular study. http://www.centerwatch.com/.

ClinicalTrials.gov

This governmental site is sponsored by the NIH and offers a wealth of information about clinical trials in general, as well as specific trials underway. Its search engine allows the user to query the database of more than 100,000 studies using a variety of methods, such as topic or geography. Online: https://www.clinicaltrials.gov/.

Coalition of Cancer Cooperative Groups

"CancerTrialsHelp.org is provided by a nonprofit coalition working to improve physician and patient access to cancer clinical trials through education, outreach, advocacy and research. Our Board Members are the leaders of the United States' publicly funded cancer cooperative clinical research program."[29] Online: http://www.cancertrialshelp.org/default.aspx.

National Cancer Institute (NCI) Clinical Trials

The NCI offers detailed information on current and past clinical trials. Its website allows you to "Search NCI's list of 12,000+ clinical trials now accepting participants, or use more search options to search the set of 25,000+ clinical trials that are no longer recruiting."[30] Online: http://www.cancer.gov/clinicaltrials/search.

World Health Organization (WHO) International Clinical Trials Registry Platform Search Portal

The WHO provides a database of worldwide clinical trials that is searchable on the website, www.who.int/trialsearch/.

HOSPICE CARE

The following organizations can provide information about hospice.[31]

National Hospice and Palliative Care Organization

1-800-658-8898 (helpline)
1-877-658-8896 (multilingual line)
caringinfo@nhpco.org
http://www.caringinfo.org

> Caring Connections began in 2004 with generous funding from the
> Robert Wood Johnson Foundation. A program of the National Hos-
> pice and Palliative Care Organization, Caring Connections works to
> ensure that individuals have access to information that informs ad-
> vance care planning, care at the end of life and the grief process.
> Caring Connections relies on philanthropic support to fund the free
> services provided to tens of thousands of individuals each year, in-
> cluding a toll free HelpLine, a multilingual HelpLine, outreach to
> traditionally under-served populations and free educational materi-
> als, including advance directives.[32]

Online: http://www.caringinfo.org/i4a/pages/index.cfm?pageid=1.

Hospice Association of America

202-546-4759
http://www.nahc.org/HAA/

The Hospice Association of America provides a variety of materials on
important hospice-related topics.

Hospice Net

info@hospicenet.org
http://www.hospicenet.org

Hospice Net is an important source of information and support for
patients with life-threatening illnesses, as well as for their families and
friends.

American Cancer Society

1-800-ACS-2345 (1-800-227-2345)
http://www.cancer.org

The American Cancer Society (ACS) provides free fact sheets and publications about hospice. The address of a local ACS chapter can be
obtained by calling the organization's toll-free telephone number.

TO FIND A COUNSELOR

American Psychosocial Oncology Society (APOS)

Toll-free number: 1-866-276-7443

Leave a message with your name, phone number(s), patient's city and
state of residence, area code of the town where you are searching for a
referral, and the patient's cancer diagnosis. They usually find someone
and call back within twenty-four to forty-eight hours. Online: www.
apos-society.org.

NOTES

PROLOGUE

1. Regina Brett, "Regina Brett Quotes," BrainyQuote, http://www.brainyquote.com/quotes/quotes/r/reginabret586752.html.

2. Anne C. Reb, "Transforming the Death Sentence: Elements of Hope in Women with Advanced Ovarian Cancer," *Oncology Nursing Forum* 73, no. 6 (2007): 73.

3. "Managing the Costs of Your Cancer Treatment," American Cancer Society, last modified August 4, 2014, http://www.cancer.org/treatment/findingandpayingfortreatment/managinginsuranceissues/the-cost-of-cancer-treatment.

4. Ibid.

5. Karen Sepucha, in discussion with the author, June 12, 2014, Cambridge, MA, by telephone.

6. Bill E., in discussion with the author, June 10, 2014, Kansas City, MO.

7. Ibid.

1. A DEFINITIVE DIAGNOSIS

1. Dana B., in discussion with the author, May 14, 2014, Overland Park, KS.

2. Diane C., in discussion with the author, June 15, 2014, Leawood, KS.

3. Steven M., in discussion with the author, May 2, 2014, Lawrence, KS.

4. Tara Parker-Pope, "Scientists Seek to Rein in Diagnoses of Cancer," *New York Times*, July 29, 2013, http://well.blogs.nytimes.com/2013/07/29/

report-suggests-sweeping-changes-to-cancer-detection-and-treatment/?
action=click&module=Search&region=searchResults%230&version=&url=
http%3A%2F%2Fquery.nytimes.com%2Fse.

5. Darrell H., in discussion with the author, June 19, 2014, Leawood, KS.

6. "Cancer Staging," National Cancer Institute, May 3, 2013, http://www.
cancer.gov/cancertopics/factsheet/detection/staging.

7. Shelley W., in discussion with the author, March 14, 2014, Kansas City,
MO.

8. Ibid.

2. HOW PROGNOSIS INFLUENCES YOUR TREATMENT

1. Shelley W., in discussion with the author, March 14, 2014, Kansas City,
MO.

2. Karen Sue Schaepe, "Bad News and First Impressions: Patient and
Family Caregiver Accounts of Learning the Cancer Diagnosis," *Social Science
in Medicine* 73, no. 6 (September 2011): 918, http://www.sciencedirect.com/
science/article/pii/S0277953611004060.

3. David E. Weissman, "Fast Fact #13: Determining Prognosis in Advanced Cancer," Center to Advance Palliative Care, last modified March 2009,
https://www.capc.org/fast-facts/13-determining-prognosis-advanced-cancer/.

4. Myra C., in discussion with the author, June 26, 2014, Kansas City, MO.

5. Linda Emanuel et al., "Clarifying Diagnosis and Prognosis in Cancer:
Guidance for Healthcare Providers," *Medscape*, March 30, 2011, http://www.
medscape.org/viewarticle/739252.

6. Moyra A. Mills and Kate Sullivan, "The Importance of Information Giving for Patients Newly Diagnosed with Cancer: A Review of the Literature,"
Journal of Clinical Nursing, no. 8 (1999): 634.

7. Ibid., 641, citing Evans, "The Experiences and Needs of Patients Attending a Cancer Support Group," *International Journal of Palliative Nursing*
1 (1995): 189–94.

8. Emanuel et al., "Clarifying Diagnosis."

9. Ibid.

10. Bill E., in discussion with the author, June 10, 2014, Kansas City, MO.

11. Thomas J. Smith et al., "A Pilot Trial of Decision Aids to Give Truthful
Prognostic and Treatment Information to Chemotherapy Patients with Advanced Cancer," *Journal of Supportive Oncology* 9, no. 2 (2011): 83, http://
www.ncbi.nlm.nih.gov/pmc/articles/PMC3589716/pdf/nihms-447553.pdf.

12. Maiko Fujimori and Yosuke Uchitomi, "Preferences of Cancer Patients
Regarding Communication of Bad News: A Systematic Literature Review,"

Japan Journal of Clinical Oncology 39, no. 4 (February 3, 2009): 213, http://
jjco.oxfordjournals.org/content/39/4/201.full.pdf.

13. Bethany J. Russell and Alicia M. Ward, "Deciding What Information Is
Necessary: Do Patients with Advanced Cancer Want to Know All the Details?"
Cancer Management and Research 3 (2011): 194.

14. Fujimori and Uchitomi, "Preferences of Cancer Patients," 213.

15. L. Furber et al., "Investigating Communication in Cancer Consultations: What Can Be Learned from Doctor and Patient Accounts of Their Experience?" *European Journal of Cancer Care* 22 (2013): 660.

16. Dana B., in discussion with the author, May 14, 2014, Overland Park,
KS.

17. Medscape, http://www.medscape.com/.

18. Sandeep Jauhar, "When Doctors Need to Lie," *New York Times*, February 22, 2014, http://www.nytimes.com/2014/02/23/opinion/sunday/when-
doctors-need-to-lie.html?_r=0.

19. Mills and Sullivan, "Importance of Information Giving," 633.

20. Furber et al., "Investigating Communication in Cancer," 657.

21. Jane E. Brody, "When Treating Cancer Is Not an Option," *New York
Times*, November 19, 2012, http://well.blogs.nytimes.com/2012/11/19/when-
treating-cancer-is-not-an-option/?_php=true&_type=blogs&_r=0.

22. Jauhar, "When Doctors Need to Lie."

23. Jennifer W. Mack and Thomas J. Smith, "Reasons Why Physicians Do
Not Have Discussions about Poor Prognosis, Why It Matters, and What Can
Be Improved," *Journal of Clinical Oncology* 30, no. 22 (August 1, 2012): 2715,
http://jco.ascopubs.org/content/30/22/2715.full.

24. Smith et al., "Pilot Trial," 1, citing C. K. Daugherty and F. J. Hlubocky,
"What Are Terminally Ill Cancer Patients Told about Their Expected Deaths?
A Study of Cancer Physicians' Self-Reports of Prognosis Disclosure," *Journal
of Clinical Oncology* 26, no. 36 (December 2008): 5988–93.

25. Ibid., 3, citing E. B. Lamont and N. A. Christakis, "Prognostic Disclosure to Patients with Cancer Near the End of Life," *Annals of Internal Medicine* 134, no. 12 (2001): 1096–1105, and P. Glare et al., "A Systematic Review
of Physicians' Survival Predictions in Terminally Ill Cancer Patients," *British
Medical Journal* 327 (2003): 195–200.

26. Mack and Smith, "Reasons Why Physicians," 2716, citing S. J. Lee et al.,
"Discrepancies between Patient and Physician Estimates for the Success of
Stem Cell Transplantation," *Journal of the American Medical Association* 285
(2001): 1034–38, and S. J. Lee et al., "Optimistic Expectations and Survival
after Hematopoietic Stem Cell Transplantation," *Biology of Blood and Marrow
Transplantation* 9 (2003): 389–96.

27. Russell and Ward, "Deciding What Information," 192, citing C. G. Koedoot et al., "The Content and Amount of Information Given by Medical Oncologists When Telling Patients with Advanced Cancer What Their Treatment Options Are: Palliative Chemotherapy and Watchful-Waiting," *European Journal of Cancer* 40, no. 2 (2004): 225–35.

28. Cornelius J. Woelk, "How Long Have I Got?" *Canadian Family Physician* 55 (December 2009): 1204.

29. Paul Glare, "Clinical Predictors of Survival in Advanced Cancer," *Journal of Supportive Oncology* 3, no. 5 (2005): 332.

30. Emanuel et al., "Clarifying Diagnosis."

31. Glare, "Clinical Predictors," 331.

32. American Cancer Society, *Cancer Facts & Figures 2014* (Atlanta: American Cancer Society, 2014), 6, http://www.cancer.org/acs/groups/content/@research/documents/webcontent/acspc-042151.pdf.

33. Ibid., 14.

34. Ibid., 15.

3. HOW TO SELECT YOUR DOCTORS AND TREATMENT FACILITIES

1. Myra C., in discussion with the author, June 26, 2014, Kansas City, MO.

2. Ibid.

3. Alta F., in discussion with the author, June 11, 2014, Kansas City, MO.

4. "How to Find a Doctor or Treatment Facility If You Have Cancer," National Cancer Institute, last modified June 5, 2013, http://www.cancer.gov/cancertopics/factsheet/Therapy/doctor-facility.

5. Malcolm Gladwell, *Outliers* (New York: Little, Brown, 2008).

6. "How to Find a Doctor."

7. "About the Cancer Centers Program," National Cancer Institute, August 13, 2012, http://www.cancer.gov/researchandfunding/extramural/cancercenters/about.

8. Ibid.

9. Myra C.

10. National Cancer Institute, "Fact Sheet."

11. "How to Find a Doctor."

12. Myra C.

4. GENETIC TESTING IN DIAGNOSIS AND TREATMENT

1. Mary E., in discussion with the author, June 18, 2014, Leawood, KS.

2. Ibid.

3. Rebecca Nagy, Kevin Sweet, and Charis Eng, "Highly Penetrant Hereditary Cancer Syndromes," *Oncogene* 23, no. 38 (2004): 6445, http://www.nature.com/onc/journal/v23/n38/full/1207714a.html.

4. Bronson D. Riley et al., "Essential Elements of Genetic Cancer Risk Assessment, Counseling, and Testing: Updated Recommendations of the National Society of Genetic Counselors," *Journal of Genetic Counseling* 21 (2012): 153.

5. Ibid.

6. "Genetic Testing: What You Need to Know," American Cancer Society, last modified October 18, 2013, http://www.cancer.org/cancer/cancercauses/geneticsandcancer/genetictesting/genetic-testing-who-should-test.

7. Mary E.

8. Associated Press, "F.D.A. Clears Cancer Test That Uses Patients' DNA," *New York Times*, August 11, 2014, http://www.nytimes.com/2014/08/12/business/fda-clears-cancer-test-that-uses-patients-dna.html.

9. Meghan L. Underhill and Cheryl B. Crotser, "Seeking Balance: Decision Support Needs of Women without Cancer and a Deleterious BRCA1 or BRCA2 Mutation," *Journal of Genetic Counseling* 23, no. 3 (November 22, 2013): 1.

10. Roni Caryn Rabin, "In Israel, a Push to Screen for Cancer Gene Leaves Many Conflicted," *New York Times*, November 26, 2011, http://www.nytimes.com/2013/11/27/health/in-israel-a-push-to-screen-for-cancer-gene-leaves-many-conflicted.html.

11. Antonis C. Antoniou et al., "Breast-Cancer Risk in Families with Mutations in PALB2," *New England Journal of Medicine*, no. 371 (August 7, 2014): 497, http://www.nejm.org/doi/full/10.1056/NEJMoa1400382.

12. Ibid.

13. "Lynch Syndrome," Genetics Home Reference, U.S. National Library of Medicine, last modified May 2013, http://ghr.nlm.nih.gov/condition/lynch-syndrome.

14. Ibid.

15. Riley et al., "Essential Elements," 156–57.

16. Mary E.

17. Kira Peikoff, "Fearing Punishment for Bad Genes," *New York Times*, April 7, 2014, http://www.nytimes.com/2014/04/08/science/fearing-punishment-for-bad-genes.html.

18. Rabin, "In Israel."

19. Christine Laronga, "Patient Information: Breast Cancer Guide to Diagnosis and Treatment (Beyond the Basics)," UpToDate, last modified September 26, 2013, http://www.uptodate.com/contents/breast-cancer-guide-to-diagnosis-and-treatment-beyond-the-basics.

20. Underhill and Crotser, "Seeking Balance."

21. Mary E.

5. MAKING SENSE OF YOUR TREATMENT OPTIONS

1. Stephen M., in discussion with the author, May 2, 2014, Lawrence, KS.

2. "After Diagnosis: A Guide for Patients and Families," American Cancer Society, last updated April 7, 2014, www.cancer.org/acs/groups/cid/documents/webcontent/002813-pdf.pdf.

3. Karen Sepucha, in discussion with the author, June 12, 2014, Cambridge, MA, by telephone.

4. Ibid.

5. Ibid.

6. Ibid.

7. Mayo Clinic Staff, "Cancer Treatment Decisions: 5 Steps to Help You Decide," Mayo Clinic, May 4, 2013, http://www.mayoclinic.org/diseases-conditions/cancer/in-depth/cancer-treatment/art-20047350.

8. Darrell H., in discussion with the author, June 19, 2014, Leawood, KS.

9. "After Diagnosis."

10. Karen Sue Schaepe, "Bad News and First Impressions: Patient and Family Caregiver Accounts of Learning the Cancer Diagnosis," *Social Science in Medicine* 73, no. 6 (September 2011): 917, http://www.sciencedirect.com/science/article/pii/S0277953611004060.

11. Inga T. Lennes et al., "Predictors of Newly Diagnosed Cancer Patients' Understanding of the Goals of Their Care at Initiation of Chemotherapy," *Cancer* (February 1, 2013): 695, http://www.ncbi.nlm.nih.gov/pmc/articles/PMC3531571/.

12. Sepucha.

13. Erin P. Balogh et al., "Patient-Centered Cancer Treatment Planning: Improving the Quality of Oncology Care. Summary of an Institute of Medicine Workshop," *The Oncologist* 16 (2011): 1800, https://theoncologist.alphamedpress.org/content/16/12/1800.full.pdf.

14. Ibid.

15. Ibid., 1801.

16. "After Diagnosis," 14.

17. John Leifer, *The Myths of Modern Medicine: The Alarming Truth about American Health Care* (Lanham, MD: Rowman and Littlefield, 2014), 75.

18. Balogh et al., "Patient-Centered Cancer Treatment Planning," 1801.

19. Ibid.

20. Ibid., 1803.

21. Yael Schenker et al., "Interventions to Improve Patient Comprehension in Informed Consent for Medical and Surgical Procedures: A Systematic Review," *Medical Decision Making* 31, no. 1 (January–February 2011): 152, http://mdm.sagepub.com/content/31/1/151.short.

22. Ibid.

23. Balogh et al., "Patient-Centered Cancer Treatment Planning," 1802.

24. Sepucha.

25. Ibid.

26. "Patient and Caregiver Resources," National Comprehensive Cancer Network, 2014, http://www.nccn.org/patients/guidelines/default.aspx.

27. Ibid.

28. Ibid.

29. Ibid.

30. Kent A. Sepkowitz, "Looking for the Final Word on Treatment," *New York Times*, May 14, 2014, http://www.nytimes.com/2014/05/14/health/looking-for-the-final-word-on-treatment.html?_r=0.

31. Ibid.

32. Nancy L. Keating et al., "Cancer Patients' Role in Clinical Decisions: Do Characteristics of the Decision Influence Roles?" *Journal of Clinical Oncology* 28, no. 28 (October 1, 2010): 4364, http://jco.ascopubs.org/content/early/2010/08/16/JCO.2009.26.8870.full.pdf.

33. Ibid.

34. Balogh et al., "Patient-Centered Cancer Treatment Planning," 1801.

35. Sally Thorne et al., "Changing Communication Needs and Preferences across the Cancer Care Trajectory: Insights from the Patient Perspective," *Supportive Care in Cancer* 22, no. 4 (April 2014), http://link.springer.com/article/10.1007/s00520-013-2056-4.

36. Steven J. Katz and Monica Morrow, "Contralateral Prophylactic Mastectomy for Breast Cancer: Addressing Peace of Mind," *The Journal of the American Medical Association* 310, no. 8 (August 28, 2013): 793–94, http://jama.jamanetwork.com/article.aspx?articleid=1723134.

37. Sepucha.

38. John Wennberg and Alan Gittelsohn, "Small Area Variations in Health Care Delivery," *Science* 182, no. 4117 (December 1973): 1102–8, doi:10.1126/science.182.4117.1102.

39. Ibid.

40. Leifer, *Myths of Modern Medicine.*

41. Ann D. Colosia et al., "A Review and Characterization of the Various Perceptions of Quality Cancer Care," *Cancer* (March 1, 2011): 891, http://www.ncbi.nlm.nih.gov/pmc/articles/PMC3073118/pdf/cncr0117-0884.pdf.

42. Ibid., 893.

6. UNDERSTANDING CLINICAL TRIALS

1. "The FDA's Drug Review Process: Ensuring Drugs Are Safe and Effective," U.S. Food and Drug Administration, last modified November 6, 2014, http://www.fda.gov/drugs/resourcesforyou/consumers/ucm143534.htm.

2. "SOAPP (Symptom Outcomes and Practice Patterns)," Eastern Cooperative Oncology Group, 2012, http://www.ecogsoapp.com/about.html.

3. Ibid.

4. Valerie Jenkins et al., "What Oncologists Believe They Said and What Patients Believe They Heard: An Analysis of Phase I Trial Discussions," *Journal of Clinical Oncology* 29, no. 1 (January 1, 2011): 61, http://jco.ascopubs.org/content/29/1/61.full.pdf.

5. "FDA's Drug Review Process."

6. Ibid.

7. Darrell H., in discussion with the author, June 19, 2014, Leawood, KS.

8. Darrell H., in e-mail to friends, April 5, 2013.

9. "About Clinical Trials," Cancer.Net, November 2013, http://www.cancer.net/print/24876.

10. Ibid.

11. "SOAPP."

12. "About Clinical Trials."

13. "Learn about Clinical Studies," ClinicalTrials.gov, last modified August 2012, http://www.clinicaltrials.gov/ct2/about-studies/learn.

14. Susan Gubar, "Living with Cancer: The New Medicine," *New York Times*, June 26, 2014, http://well.blogs.nytimes.com/2014/06/26/living-with-cancer-the-new-medicine/.

7. THE IMPORTANCE OF GETTING A SECOND OPINION

1. "How to Find a Doctor or Treatment Facility If You Have Cancer," National Cancer Institute, 2013, http://www.cancer.gov/cancertopics/factsheet/Therapy/doctor-facility.

2. Jennifer Philip et al., "Second Medical Opinions: The Views of Oncology Patients and Their Physicians," *Supportive Care in Cancer* 18, no. 9 (September 2010): 1203, http://www.ncbi.nlm.nih.gov/pubmed/19802635.

3. Shelley W. in discussion with the author, March 14, 2014, Leawood, KS.

4. Laurie Tarkan, "Value of Second Opinions Is Underscored in Study of Biopsies," *New York Times*, April 4, 2000, http://www.nytimes.com/2000/04/04/health/value-of-second-opinions-is-underscored-in-study-of-biopsies.html.

5. Marc Beishon, "A Second Opinion, Because There's No Second Chance," *Cancer World* (January/February 2007): 15, http://www.cancerworld.org/pdf/8775_CW16_14-19_GrandroundOK.pdf.

6. Philip et al., "Second Medical Opinions," 1203.

7. Ibid., 1199.

8. Ibid.

9. Darrell H., in discussion with the author, June 19, 2014, Leawood, KS.

8. THE EMOTIONAL ROLLER COASTER OF CANCER

1. Wolfgang Linden et al., "Anxiety and Depression after Cancer Diagnosis: Prevalence Rates by Cancer Type, Gender, and Age," *Journal of Affective Disorders* 141, nos. 2–3 (December 10, 2012): 343, http://www.sciencedirect.com/science/article/pii/S0165032712002212.

2. Dana B., in discussion with the author, May 14, 2014, Leawood, KS.

3. "Distress in People with Cancer," American Cancer Society, last modified August 13, 2014, http://www.cancer.org/acs/groups/cid/documents/webcontent/002827-pdf.pdf.

4. Linden et al., "Anxiety and Depression," 344.

5. Karlynn M. Brintzenhofe-Szoc et al., "Mixed Anxiety/Depression Symptoms in a Large Cancer Cohort: Prevalence by Cancer Type," *Psychosomatics* 50, no. 4 (July–August 2009): 384, http://www.sciencedirect.com/science/article/pii/S0033318209708230.

6. Linden et al., "Anxiety and Depression," 343.

7. Allison W. Boyes et al., "Flourishing or Floundering? Prevalence and Correlates of Anxiety and Depression among a Population-Based Sample of Adult Cancer Survivors 6 Months after Diagnosis," *Journal of Affective Disorders* 135, nos. 1–3 (December 2011): 185, http://www.ncbi.nlm.nih.gov/pubmed/21864913.

8. Linden et al., "Anxiety and Depression," 343.

9. A. Hinz et al., "Anxiety and Depression in Cancer Patients Compared with the General Population," *European Journal of Cancer Care* 19, no. 4 (July 2010): 527, http://onlinelibrary.wiley.com/doi/10.1111/j.1365-2354.2009.

01088.x/abstract?systemMessage=Wiley+Online+Library+will+be+disrupted+
Saturday%2C+15+March+from+10%3A00-12%3A00+GMT+%2806%3A00-
08%3A00+EDT%29+for+essential+maintenance.

10. Alex J. Mitchell et al., "Meta-analysis of Screening and Case Finding
Tools for Depression in Cancer: Evidence Based Recommendations for Clinical Practice on Behalf of the Depression in Cancer Care Consensus Group,"
Journal of Affective Disorders 140, no. 2 (October 2012): 150, http://www.
sciencedirect.com/science/article/pii/S0165032711008068.

11. Laura Landro, "To Treat the Cancer, Treat the Distress," *Wall Street
Journal*, August 27, 2012, http://online.wsj.com/news/articles/
SB10000872396390444914904577615291424503430.

12. Isabelle Merckaert et al., "Cancer Patients' Desire for Psychological
Support: Prevalence and Implications for Screening Patients' Psychological
Needs," *Psycho-Oncology* 19, no. 2 (February 2010): 141, http://onlinelibrary.
wiley.com/doi/10.1002/pon.1568/pdf.

13. Landro, "To Treat the Cancer."

14. Mitchell et al., "Meta-analysis of Screening," 150.

15. Paul Glare, "Clinical Predictors of Survival in Advanced Cancer," *Journal of Supportive Oncology* 3, no. 5 (2005): 335.

16. Ibid.

17. Moira Mulhern, in discussion with the author, August 27, 2014, Leawood, KS.

18. Landro, "To Treat the Cancer."

19. "Distress in People with Cancer."

20. Ibid.

21. Melissa Etheridge, "Melissa Etheridge Quotes," BrainyQuote, http://
www.brainyquote.com/quotes/authors/m/melissa_etheridge_2.html.

22. Anna Casellas-Grau, Antoni Font, and Jaume Vives, "Positive Psychology Interventions in Breast Cancer: A Systematic Review, *Psycho-Oncology* 23,
no. 1 (2014): 10, http://onlinelibrary.wiley.com/doi/10.1002/pon.3353/pdf.

23. Bill E., in discussion with the author, June 10, 2014, Kansas City, MO.

24. Mulhern.

9. METHODS TO MINIMIZE SIDE EFFECTS

1. Ali H., in discussion with the author, August 15, 2014, Leawood, KS.

2. Ann M. Berger, Lynn H. Gerber, and Deborah K. Mayer, "Cancer-
Related Fatigue," *Journal of National Comprehensive Cancer Network* 8, no. 8
(August 1, 2010): 904–31, http://www.jnccn.org/content/8/8/904.short.

3. Ibid., 904.

4. Markus Horneber et al., "Cancer-Related Fatigue: Epidemiology, Pathogenesis, Diagnosis, and Treatment," *Deutsches Arzteblatt International* 109, no. 9 (2012): 162, http://www.aerzteblatt.de/int/archive/article/122875/Cancer-Related-Fatigue-Epidemiology-Pathogenesis-Diagnosis-and-Treatment.

5. Ibid.

6. Ibid., 166.

7. Dana B., in discussion with the author, May 14, 2014, Overland Park, KS.

8. Bill E., in discussion with the author, June 10, 2014, Kansas City, MO.

9. Diane C., in discussion with the author, June 25, 2014, Leawood, KS.

10. Matthew Stenger, "Nurse Navigators Improve Patient-Reported Quality of Care in Early Cancer Care," ASCO Post, December 3, 2013, http://www.ascopost.com/ViewNews.aspx?nid=10799.

11. Andrew Pollack, "Drug Saves Fertility for Women with Cancer," *New York Times*, May 30, 2014, http://www.nytimes.com/2014/05/31/business/drug-could-protect-fertility-in-breast-cancer-patients.html.

10. MAKE NUTRITION AND EXERCISE PART OF YOUR TREATMENT PLAN

1. Ali H., in discussion with the author, August 15, 2014, Leawood, KS.

2. "Nutrition in Cancer Care (PDQ)," National Cancer Institute, last modified December 5, 2014, http://www.cancer.gov/cancertopics/pdq/supportivecare/nutrition/Patient/page4.

3. Ibid.

4. Bill E., in discussion with the author, June 10, 2014, Kansas City, MO.

5. "Nutrition for the Person with Cancer during Treatment: A Guide for Patients and Families," American Cancer Society, last modified June 9, 2014, 6, http://www.cancer.org/acs/groups/cid/documents/webcontent/002903-pdf.pdf.

6. Ibid.

7. "Nutrition in Cancer Care."

8. Ibid.

9. Ibid.

10. Ibid.

11. Ibid.

12. "Nutrition for the Person with Cancer," 10.

13. "Guidelines Urge Exercise for Cancer Patients, Survivors," *National Cancer Institute (NCI) Cancer Bulletin* 7, no. 3 (June 29, 2010).

14. Victoria Mock et al., "Fatigue and Quality of Life Outcomes of Exercise during Cancer Treatment," *Cancer Practice* 9, no. 3 (May/June 2001), 120.

15. "Trim Your Cancer Risk with Exercise," Fred Hutchinson Cancer Research Center, 2015, https://www.fhcrc.org/en/events/healthy-living/Trim-Risk.html.

16. Ibid., 1415.

17. "Guidelines Urge Exercise," 2.

11. WHAT TO EXPECT FROM PAIN CONTROL

1. "Pain Management," Stanford Health Care, 2015, https://stanfordhealthcare.org/medical-conditions/pain/cancer-pain.html.

2. "Pain Management—Pain Management," Community Health Network, n.d., http://www.ecommunity.com/health/index.aspx?pageID=P07302.

3. "Pain (PDQ)," National Cancer Institute, last updated April 10, 2014, http://www.cancer.gov/cancertopics/pdq/supportivecare/pain/Patient/page1/AllPages.

4. "Pain Management—Pain Management."

5. "Pain (PDQ)."

6. "Pain Management."

7. "Pain (PDQ)."

8. Ibid.

9. Ibid.

10. Ibid.

11. Judy Foreman, *A Nation in Pain: Healing Our Biggest Health Problem* (Oxford, UK: Oxford University Press, 2014).

12. HOW TO MANAGE THE COST OF CANCER

1. Jeffrey Nadel and Kavita Patel, "Changing the Way We Pay for Cancer Care," Brookings Institute, June 9, 2014, http://www.brookings.edu/research/opinions/2014/06/09-cancer-care-payment-reform-patel.

2. American Cancer Society, *Cancer Facts & Figures 2014* (Atlanta: American Cancer Society, 2014), 3, http://www.cancer.org/acs/groups/content/@research/documents/webcontent/acspc-042151.pdf.

3. "Biggest Cause of Personal Bankruptcy: Medical Bills," Today, June 25, 2013, http://www.today.com/money/biggest-cause-personal-bankruptcy-medical-bills-6C10442408.

4. Julia S., in discussion with the author, June 12, 2014, Kansas City, MO.

5. Ibid.

6. Rhonda C., in discussion with the author, September 16, 2014, Kansas City, MO.

7. S. Yousuf Zafar, "How Should We Assess and Address the Financial Toxicity of Cancer Care?" *ASCO Connection*, April 22, 2014, http://connection.asco.org/Magazine/Article/ID/3849/Cost-of-Cancer-Care-A-Crucial-Physician-Patient-Conversation.aspx.

8. Ibid.

9. Rhonda C.

10. Jennifer Mellace, "The Financial Burden of Cancer Care," *Social Work Today* 10, no. 2 (March/April 2010): 14, http://www.socialworktoday.com/archive/032210p14.shtml.

11. Julia S.

12. Ann D. Colosia et al., "A Review and Characterization of the Various Perceptions of Quality Cancer Care," *Cancer* (March 1, 2011), 888, http://www.ncbi.nlm.nih.gov/pmc/articles/PMC3073118/pdf/cncr0117-0884.pdf.

13. Julia S.

14. Ibid.

15. Rhonda C.

16. Andrew Pollack, "Doctors Denounce Cancer Drug Prices of $100,000 a Year," *New York Times*, April 25, 2013, http://www.nytimes.com/2013/04/26/business/cancer-physicians-attack-high-drug-costs.html.

17. Ibid.

18. Hagop Kantarjian, "The Price of Drugs for Chronic Myeloid Leukemia (CML); A Reflection of the Unsustainable Prices of Cancer Drugs: From the Perspective of a Large Group of CML Experts," *Blood* (April 25, 2013): 9, http://bloodjournal.hematologylibrary.org/content/early/2013/04/23/blood-2013-03-490003.full.pdf.

19. Kjel Johnson et al., *Innovation in Cancer Care and Implications for Health Systems: Global Oncology Trend Report* (Plymouth Meeting, PA: IMS Institute for Healthcare Informatics, 2014), 1, http://www.imshealth.com/portal/site/imshealth/menuitem.762a961826aad98f53c753c71ad8c22a/?vgnextoid=f8d4df7a5e8b5410VgnVCM10000076192ca2RCRD.

20. Kantarjian, "Price of Drugs," 5.

21. Johnson et al., *Innovation in Cancer Care*, 3.

22. Ibid., 14.

23. Kantarjian, "Price of Drugs," 4.

24. Nadel and Patel, "Changing the Way."

25. "Managing the Costs of Your Cancer Treatment," American Cancer Society, last updated August 4, 2014, http://www.cancer.org/treatment/

findingandpayingfortreatment/managinginsuranceissues/the-cost-of-cancer-treatment.

26. Julia S.

27. "Managing the Costs."

13. WHEN CONSIDERING COMPLEMENTARY THERAPIES

1. Mary E., in discussion with the author, June 18, 2014, Leawood, KS.

2. Joel G. Anderson and Ann Gill Taylor, "Use of Complementary Therapies for Cancer Symptom Management: Results of the 2007 National Health Interview Survey," *Journal of Alternative and Complementary Medicine* 18, no. 3 (March 2012): 235, http://www.ncbi.nlm.nih.gov/pmc/articles/PMC3306580/.

3. Ibid.

4. Edzard Ernst, "Alternative Treatments for Breast Cancer," *European Journal of Clinical Pharmacology* 68 (2012): 453, http://paperity.org/p/19734319/alternative-treatments-for-breast-cancer.

5. Gabriel Miller, Barrie R. Cassileth, and Edzard Ernst, "Asking the Experts: Complementary and Alternative Medicine and Cancer," Medscape, September 2, 2014, http://www.medscape.com/viewarticle/830553.

6. Peter J. Smith et al., "Why Do Some Cancer Patients Receiving Chemotherapy Choose to Take Complementary and Alternative Medicines and What Are the Risks?" *Asia-Pacific Journal of Clinical Oncology* 10, no. 1 (March 2014): 2, http://onlinelibrary.wiley.com/doi/10.1111/ajco.12115/abstract;jsessionid=B9CC99FF876B420DF4063ADC14921E51.f04t02?systemMessage=Wiley+Online+Library+will+be+disrupted+Saturday%2C+15+March+from+10%3A00-12%3A00+GMT+%2806%3A00-08%3A00+EDT%29+for+essential+maintenance.

7. Jun James Mao et al., "Complementary and Alternative Medicine Use among Cancer Survivors: A Population-Based Study," *Journal of Cancer Survivorship* 5, no. 1 (March 2011): 8–9, http://www.ncbi.nlm.nih.gov/pmc/articles/PMC3564962/pdf/nihms-438873.pdf.

8. Adam Perlman et al., "Prevalence and Correlates of Postdiagnosis Initiation of Complementary and Alternative Medicine among Patients at a Comprehensive Cancer Center," *Journal of Oncology Practice* 9, no. 1 (January 2013): 35, http://www.ncbi.nlm.nih.gov/pmc/articles/PMC3545661/pdf/jop34.pdf.

9. Anderson and Taylor, "Use of Complementary Therapies," 236.

10. Perlman et al., "Prevalence and Correlates," 34.

11. "Cancer and CAM: What the Science Says," *NCCAM Clinical Digest* (October 2010), 3.

12. Mary E.

13. Smith et al., "Cancer Patients Receiving Chemotherapy," 3.

14. Perlman et al., "Prevalence and Correlates," 34.

15. Anderson and Taylor, "Use of Complementary Therapies," 239.

16. Smith et al., "Cancer Patients Receiving Chemotherapy," 4.

17. Miller, Cassileth, and Ernst, "Asking the Experts."

18. William T. Jarvis, "Cancer Quackery," National Council against Health Fraud (December 17, 2000), http://www.ncahf.org/articles/c-d/caquackery.html.

19. Ibid.

20. "Medicine: Cancer Quacks," *Time*, February 28, 1955, http://content.time.com/time/magazine/article/0,9171,861227,00.html.

21. David Gorski, "Another Cancer Tragedy in the Making," *Science-Based Medicine*, May 14, 2012, http://www.sciencebasedmedicine.org/another-cancer-tragedy-in-the-making/.

22. Ibid.

23. Smith et al., "Cancer Patients Receiving Chemotherapy," 3.

24. "Royal Rife," Wikipedia, http://en.wikipedia.org/wiki/Royal_Rife.

25. Ibid.

26. Ibid.

27. Ibid.

28. Ibid.

29. Jarvis, "Cancer Quackery."

30. Ibid.

31. Ibid.

32. Ibid.

33. Mao et al., "Complementary and Alternative Medicine," 12.

14. THE ROLE OF YOUR CAREGIVERS

1. Dana B., in discussion with the author, May 14, 2014, Overland Park, KS.

2. Dana B.

3. Ibid.

4. "What You Need to Know as a Cancer Caregiver," American Cancer Society, last modified April 28, 2014, 1, http://www.cancer.org/acs/groups/cid/documents/webcontent/acspc-027595-pdf.pdf.

5. Diane C., in discussion with the author, June 25, 2014, Leawood, KS.

6. Ibid.

7. "What You Need to Know," 5.

8. Ibid.

9. Ibid.

10. Laurel L. Northouse et al., "Interventions with Family Caregivers of Cancer Patients: Meta-Analysis of Randomized Trials," *CA: A Cancer Journal for Clinicians* 60, no. 5 (2010): 317, http://www.ncbi.nlm.nih.gov/pmc/articles/PMC2946584/pdf/nihms208009.pdf.

11. "What You Need to Know," 2.

12. Diane C.

13. Northouse et al., "Interventions," 318.

14. Ibid., 317.

15. Darrell H., in discussion with the author, June 19, 2014, Leawood, KS.

16. Northouse et al., "Interventions," 317.

17. "What You Need to Know," 1.

18. Northouse et al., "Interventions," 318.

19. Ibid., 337.

20. Ibid., 318.

21. Dana B.

22. "What You Need to Know," 6.

23. Shelley W., in discussion with the author, March 14, 2014, Kansas City, MO.

24. Myra C., in discussion with the author, June 26, 2014, Kansas City, MO.

15. WHEN INITIAL TREATMENT PROVES INSUFFICIENT

1. Elizabeth Edwards, "Elizabeth Edwards Quotes," BrainyQuote, http://www.brainyquote.com/quotes/authors/e/elizabeth_edwards.html.

2. Diane C., in discussion with the author, June 25, 2014, Leawood, KS.

3. Darrell H., in discussion with the author, June 19, 2014, Leawood, KS.

4. Susan Gubar, "Living with Cancer: Chronic, Not Cured," *New York Times*, June 5, 2014, http://well.blogs.nytimes.com/2014/06/05/living-with-cancer-chronic-not-cured/?_r=0.

5. Darrell H.

16. THE CHALLENGES OF SURVIVING CANCER

1. Dana B., in discussion with the author, May 14, 2014, Overland Park, KS.

2. Dave Pelzer, "Dave Pelzer Quotes," BrainyQuote, http://www.brainyquote.com/quotes/authors/d/dave_pelzer.html.

3. Regina Brett, "Regina Brett Quotes," BrainyQuote, http://www.brainyquote.com/quotes/quotes/r/reginabret586752.html.

4. Kylie Minogue, "Kylie Minogue Quotes," BrainyQuote, http://www.brainyquote.com/quotes/authors/k/kylie_minogue.html.

5. Alyssa G. Rieber, "How Being a Cancer Survivor Affects My Oncology Practice," *ASCO Connection*, April 22, 2014, http://connection.asco.org/Magazine/Article/ID/3852/How-Being-a-Cancer-Survivor-Affects-My-Oncology-Practice.aspx.

6. Nada F. Khan, Peter W. Rose, and Julie Evans, "Defining Cancer Survivorship: A More Transparent Approach Is Needed," *Journal of Cancer Survivorship* 6, no. 33 (2012): 33–34, http://link.springer.com/article/10.1007%2Fs11764-011-0194-6.

7. Patricia I. Documet et al., "Breast Cancer Survivors' Perception of Survivorship," *Oncology Nursing Forum* 39, no. 3 (May 1, 2012): 314, http://www.ncbi.nlm.nih.gov/pmc/articles/PMC3437916/pdf/nihms398533.pdf.

8. Eva Grunfeld and Craig C. Earle, "The Interface between Primary and Oncology Specialty Care: Treatment through Survivorship," *Journal of the National Cancer Institute Monographs* 40 (2010): 25, http://jncimonographs.oxfordjournals.org/content/2010/40/25.full.pdf+html.

9. Rebecca Cowens-Alvarado et al., "Advancing Survivorship Care through the National Cancer Survivorship Resource Center: Developing American Cancer Society Guidelines for Primary Care Providers," *CA: A Cancer Journal for Clinicians* 63, no. 3 (May/June 2013): 147, http://onlinelibrary.wiley.com/doi/10.3322/caac.21183/pdf.

10. Anne C. Reb, "Transforming the Death Sentence: Elements of Hope in Women with Advanced Ovarian Cancer," *Oncology Nursing Forum* 73, no. 6 (2007): 74.

11. Grunfeld and Earle, "Interface," 25.

12. Ibid.

13. Manuel Valdivieso et al., "Cancer Survivors in the United States: A Review of the Literature and a Call to Action," *International Journal of Medical Sciences* 9, no. 2 (2012): 164, http://www.ncbi.nlm.nih.gov/pmc/articles/PMC3264952/pdf/ijmsv09p0163.pdf.

14. American Cancer Society, *Cancer Facts & Figures 2014* (Atlanta: American Cancer Society, 2014), http://www.cancer.org/acs/groups/content/@research/documents/webcontent/acspc-042151.pdf.

15. Ibid., 1.

16. Ibid.

17. Rebecca Siegel et al., "Cancer Treatment and Survivorship Statistics," *CA: A Cancer Journal for Clinicians* 62, no. 4 (July/August 2012): 222, http://onlinelibrary.wiley.com/doi/10.3322/caac.21149/pdf.

18. Ibid., 223.

19. Allison W. Boyes et al., "Flourishing or Floundering? Prevalence and Correlates of Anxiety and Depression among a Population-Based Sample of Adult Cancer Survivors 6 Months after Diagnosis," *Journal of Affective Disorders* 135, nos. 1–3 (December 2011): 185, http://www.ncbi.nlm.nih.gov/pubmed/21864913.

20. Dana B.

21. Ibid.

22. Ibid.

23. Ibid.

24. Boyes et al., "Flourishing or Floundering?" 189.

25. Bruce Feiler, "Cancer Survivors Celebrate Their Cancerversary," *New York Times*, December 8, 2013, http://www.nytimes.com/2013/12/08/fashion/Cancer-Survivors-five-year-Celebration-Day-known-as-cancerversary.html?_r=0.

26. Dana B.

27. Valdivieso et al., "Cancer Survivors," 168.

28. Grunfeld and Earle, "Interface," 25.

29. Ibid.

30. Cowens-Alvarado et al., "Advancing Survivorship Care," 148.

31. Carrie N. Klabunde et al., "Physician Roles in the Cancer-Related Follow-Up Care of Cancer Survivors," *Family Medicine* 45, no. 7 (2013): 469, http://europepmc.org/articles/PMC3755767?pdf=render.

32. Arnold L. Potosky et al., "Differences between Primary Care Physicians' and Oncologists' Knowledge, Attitudes and Practices Regarding the Care of Cancer Survivors," *Journal of General Internal Medicine* 26, no. 12 (December 2011): 1406, http://link.springer.com/article/10.1007/s11606-011-1808-4#page-1.

33. Ibid., 1409.

34. Ibid., 1403.

35. Ibid., 1409.

36. Cowens-Alvarado et al., "Advancing Survivorship Care," 148.

37. Ibid.

38. Ibid., 149.

39. Documet et al., "Breast Cancer Survivors' Perception," 315.

17. DIFFICULT DECISIONS AT THE END OF THE JOURNEY

1. Darrell H., in discussion with the author, June 19, 2014, Leawood, KS.

2. Darrell H., in e-mail to friends March 4, 2013.

3. "Palliative Care in Cancer," National Cancer Institute, last modified March 16, 2010, http://www.cancer.gov/cancertopics/factsheet/Support/palliative-care.

4. Bruce J. Roth et al., "Clinical Cancer Advances 2012: Annual Report on Progress against Cancer from the American Society of Clinical Oncology," *Journal of Clinical Oncology* 31, no. 1 (January 1, 2013): 154.

5. "Palliative Care."

6. Ibid.

7. Roth et al., "Clinical Cancer Advances," 152.

8. Emanuel et al., "Clarifying Diagnosis and Prognosis in Cancer: Guidance for Healthcare Providers," *Medscape* (March 30, 2011), http://www.medscape.org/viewarticle/739252.

9. Ibid.

10. Jane E. Brody, "When Treating Cancer Is Not an Option," *New York Times*, November 19, 2012, http://well.blogs.nytimes.com/2012/11/19/when-treating-cancer-is-not-an-option/?_php=true&_type=blogs&_r=0.

11. Bethany J. Russell and Alicia M. Ward, "Deciding What Information Is Necessary: Do Patients with Advanced Cancer Want to Know All the Details?" *Cancer Management and Research* 3 (2011): 194.

12. Thomas J. Smith et al., "A Pilot Trial of Decision Aids to Give Truthful Prognostic and Treatment Information to Chemotherapy Patients with Advanced Cancer," *Journal of Supportive Oncology* 9, no. 2 (2011): 5, http://www.ncbi.nlm.nih.gov/pmc/articles/PMC3589716/pdf/nihms-447553.pdf.

13. Jennifer W. Mack and Thomas J. Smith, "Reasons Why Physicians Do Not Have Discussions about Poor Prognosis, Why It Matters, and What Can Be Improved," *Journal of Clinical Oncology* 30, no. 22 (August 1, 2012): 2716, http://jco.ascopubs.org/content/30/22/2715.full.

14. Rebecca G. Hagerty et al., "Communicating with Realism and Hope: Incurable Cancer Patients' Views on the Disclosure of Prognosis," *Journal of Clinical Oncology* 23, no. 6 (February 20, 2005): 1278, http://jco.ascopubs.org/content/23/6/1278.full.pdf.

15. Brody, "When Treating Cancer."

18. CHOOSING TO STOP TREATMENT AND THE ROLE OF HOSPICE

1. Randy Pausch, "Randy Pausch's Web Site," Carnegie Mellon University, http://www.cs.cmu.edu/~pausch/.

2. Darrell H., in discussion with the author, June 19, 2014, Leawood, KS.

3. "History of Hospice Care," National Hospice and Palliative Care Organization, http://www.nhpco.org/history-hospice-care.

4. Ibid.

5. Ibid.

6. "NHPCO's Facts and Figures: Hospice Care in America," National Hospice and Palliative Care Organization, 2013, 4, http://www.nhpco.org/sites/default/files/public/Statistics_Research/2013_Facts_Figures.pdf.

7. Ibid.

8. John Leifer, *The Myths of Modern Medicine: The Alarming Truth about American Health Care* (Lanham, MD: Rowman and Littlefield, 2014).

9. Elisabeth Kübler-Ross, *On Death and Dying* (New York: Scribner, 1969).

10. Diane C., in discussion with the author, June 25, 2014, Leawood, KS.

11. "End-of-Life Care for People Who Have Cancer," National Cancer Institute, last modified May 10, 2012, http://www.cancer.gov/cancertopics/factsheet/Support/end-of-life-care.

12. Darrell H., discussion.

13. "NHPCO's Facts and Figures," 3.

14. Ibid., 11.

15. "Nearly One Third of Medicare Patients with Advanced Cancer Die in Hospitals and ICUs; About Half Get Hospice Care," Dartmouth Institute for Health Policy and Clinical Practice, November 16, 2010, 1, http://www.dartmouthatlas.org/downloads/press/Cancer_report_release_111610.pdf.

16. "The Right Care at the Right Time: Hospice Length of Stay," Hospice Action Network, 2014, http://hospiceactionnetwork.org/linked_documents/get_informed/policy_resources/PolicyBriefing_LengthofStay_March2014.pdf.

17. Jane E. Brody, "When Treating Cancer Is Not an Option," *New York Times*, November 19, 2012, http://well.blogs.nytimes.com/2012/11/19/when-treating-cancer-is-not-an-option/?_php=true&_type=blogs&_r=0.

18. "Nearly One Third," 1.

19. "End-of-Life Care."

20. Paula Span, "When Advance Directives Are Ignored," *New York Times*, June 24, 2014, http://newoldage.blogs.nytimes.com/2014/06/24/when-advance-directives-are-ignored/.

21. Darrell H., discussion.

22. Paula Span, "How to Choose a Hospice," *New York Times*, June 17, 2014, http://newoldage.blogs.nytimes.com/2014/06/17/how-to-choose-a-hospice/.

23. Ibid.

24. Susan Gubar, "Living with Cancer: A Tour of Hospice," *New York Times*, July 24, 2014, http://well.blogs.nytimes.com/2014/07/24/living-with-cancer-a-tour-of-hospice/.

25. Thomas J. Smith et al., "A Pilot Trial of Decision Aids to Give Truthful Prognostic and Treatment Information to Chemotherapy Patients with Advanced Cancer," *Journal of Supportive Oncology* 9, no. 2 (2011), 79, http://www.ncbi.nlm.nih.gov/pmc/articles/PMC3589716/pdf/nihms-447553.pdf.

26. Ibid.

27. "End-of-Life Care."

28. Ibid.

29. Brody, "When Treating Cancer."

30. "End-of-Life Care."

31. Darrell H., discussion.

32. Darrell H., e-mail to friends, November 1, 2013.

33. Darrell H., e-mail to friends, February 25, 2014.

34. Darrell H., discussion.

35. Ibid.

36. Ibid.

37. Diane C.

38. Elisabeth Kübler-Ross, in discussion with the author, September 4, 1997, Carefree, AZ.

39. Sonja Sherry Hickey, "Enabling Hope," *Cancer Nursing* 9, no. 3 (1986): 133–37.

RESOURCES

1. "Patient and Caregiver Resources," National Comprehensive Cancer Network, 2014, http://www.nccn.org/patients/advocacy/default.aspx.

2. "About the Alliance of Dedicated Cancer Centers," Alliance of Dedicated Cancer Centers, 2011, http://www.aodcc.org/AboutADCC.aspx.

3. "AACR Mission," American Association for Cancer Research, http://www.aacr.org/aboutus/Pages/default.aspx#.VMuYNUfF9oN.

4. Ibid.

5. "ASCO Profile and Mission Statement," American Society of Clinical Oncology, 2015, http://www.asco.org/about-asco/asco-profile-and-mission-statement.

6. "Patient-Centered Sites," Association of Cancer Online Resources, 2015, http://www.acor.org/pages/resources.

7. "About the Association of Community Cancer Centers," Association of Community Cancer Centers, 2015, http://www.accc-cancer.org/about/.

8. "AOSW Mission Statement," Association of Oncology Social Work, 2014, http://www.aosw.org/aosw/Main/About-AOSW/Mission-and-Goals/AOSWMain/About-AOSW/mission-and-goals.aspx?hkey=782e2be0-de81-4c24-af6d-36c11e7bca43.

9. "Welcome," Bone and Cancer Foundation, 2011, http://www.boneandcancerfoundation.org/.

10. "About Us," CancerCare, 2015, http://www.cancercare.org/about.

11. "Cancer Experience Registry," Cancer Support Community, 2014, https://csc.cancerexperienceregistry.org/.

12. Cancer Hope Network, http://www.cancerhopenetwork.org/.

13. Cancer.net, 2015, http://www.cancer.net/.

14. "Food for Life: Cancer Project," Physicians Committee for Responsible Medicine, http://pcrm.org/health/cancer-resources.

15. "About the Cancer Support Community," Cancer Support Community, 2014, http://www.cancersupportcommunity.org/MainMenu/About-CSC/Who-We-Are.html.

16. "Cancer Symptoms, Signs and Prevention," CancerSymptoms.org, 2013, http://www.cancersymptoms.org/.

17. "About Us," CURE, 2014, http://www.curetoday.com/about-us.

18. "Where the Money Goes," LiveStrong Foundation, http://www.livestrong.org/what-we-do/our-approach/where-the-money-goes/.

19. "NCI Mission Statement," National Cancer Institute, http://www.cancer.gov/aboutnci/overview/mission.

20. "NCCIH Facts-at-a-Glance and Mission," National Center for Complementary and Integrative Health, last modified January 9, 2015, https://nccih.nih.gov/about/ataglance.

21. "NCCS Mission," National Coalition for Cancer Survivorship, 2015, http://www.canceradvocacy.org/about-us/our-mission/.

22. "About NCCN," National Comprehensive Cancer Network, 2015, http://www.nccn.org/about/default.aspx.

23. "About NHPCO," National Hospice and Palliative Care Organization, http://www.nhpco.org/about-nhpco.

24. "About NORD," National Organization for Rare Disorders, 2015, http://www.rarediseases.org/about.

25. "About ONS," Oncology Nursing Society, 2014, www.ons.org/about.

26. "Our History and Mission," Patient Advocate Foundation, 2012, http://www.patientadvocate.org/about.php?p=906.

27. "What We Do," Prevent Cancer Foundation, http://preventcancer.org/what-we-do/.

28. "About CenterWatch," CenterWatch, 2015, http://www.centerwatch.com/about-centerwatch/.

29. Coalition of Cancer Cooperative Groups, 2013, http://www.cancertrialshelp.org/default.aspx.

30. "Search for Clinical Trials," National Cancer Institute, http://www.cancer.gov/clinicaltrials/search.

31. "Hospice Care," National Cancer Institute, last modified October 25, 2012, http://www.cancer.gov/cancertopics/factsheet/Support/hospice.

32. "About Us," Caring Connections, http://www.caringinfo.org/i4a/pages/index.cfm?pageid=3401.

BIBLIOGRAPHY

"AACR Mission." American Association for Cancer Research. http://www.aacr.org/aboutus/Pages/default.aspx#.VMuYNUfF9oN.

"About CenterWatch." CenterWatch. 2015. http://www.centerwatch.com/about-centerwatch/.

"About Clinical Trials." Cancer.Net. November 2013. http://www.cancer.net/print/24876.

"About NCCN." National Comprehensive Cancer Network. 2015. http://www.nccn.org/about/default.aspx.

"About NHPCO." National Hospice and Palliative Care Organization. http://www.nhpco.org/about-nhpco.

"About NORD." National Organization for Rare Disorders. 2015. http://www.rarediseases.org/about.

"About ONS." Oncology Nursing Society. 2014. www.ons.org/about.

"About the Alliance of Dedicated Cancer Centers." Alliance of Dedicated Cancer Centers. 2011. http://www.aodcc.org/AboutADCC.aspx.

"About the Association of Community Cancer Centers." Association of Community Cancer Centers. 2015. http://www.accc-cancer.org/about/.

"About the Cancer Centers Program." National Cancer Institute. August 13, 2012. http://www.cancer.gov/researchandfunding/extramural/cancercenters/about.

"About the Cancer Support Community." Cancer Support Community. 2014. http://www.cancersupportcommunity.org/MainMenu/About-CSC/Who-We-Are.html.

"About Us." CancerCare. 2015. http://www.cancercare.org/about.

"About Us." Caring Connections. http://www.caringinfo.org/i4a/pages/index.cfm?pageid=3401.

"About Us." CURE. 2014. http://www.curetoday.com/about-us.

"After Diagnosis: A Guide for Patients and Families." American Cancer Society. Last modified April 7, 2014. http://www.cancer.org/acs/groups/cid/documents/webcontent/002813-pdf.pdf.

American Cancer Society. *Cancer Facts & Figures 2014.* Atlanta: American Cancer Society, 2014. http://www.cancer.org/acs/groups/content/@research/documents/webcontent/acspc-042151.pdf.

Anderson, Joel G., and Ann Gill Taylor. "Use of Complementary Therapies for Cancer Symptom Management: Results of the 2007 National Health Interview Survey." *Journal of Alternative and Complementary Medicine* 18, no. 3 (March 2012): 235–41. http://www.ncbi.nlm.nih.gov/pmc/articles/PMC3306580/.

Antoniou, Antonis C., Silvia Casadei, Tuomas Heikkinen, Daniel Barrowdale, Katri Pylkas, Jonathan Roberts, Andrew Lee, Deepak Subramanian, Kim De Leeneer, Florentia Fostira, Eva Tomiak, Susan L. Neuhausen, Zhi L. Teo, Sofia Khan, Kristina Attomaki, Jukka S. Moilanen, Clare Turnbull, Sheila Seal, Arto Mannermaa, Anne Kallionemi, Geoffrey J. Lindeman, Saundra S. Buys, Irene L. Andrulis, Paolo Radice, Carlo Tondini, Siranoush Manoukian, Amanda E. Toland, Penelope Miron, Jeffrey N. Weitzel, Susan M. Domcheck, Bruce Poppe, Kathleen B. M. Claes, Drakoulis Yannoukakos, Patrick Concannon, Jonine L. Bernstein, Paul A. James, Douglas F. Easton, David E. Goldgar, John L. Hopper, Nazneen Rahman, Paolo Peterlongo, Heli Neveanlinna, Mary-Claire King, Fergus J. Couch, Melissa C. Southey, Robert Winqvist, William D. Foulkes, and Marc Tischkowitz. "Breast-Cancer Risk in Families with Mutations in PALB2." *New England Journal of Medicine*, no. 371 (August 7, 2014): 497–506. www.nejm.org/doi/full/10.1056/NEJMoa1400382.

"AOSW Mission Statement." Association of Oncology Social Work. 2014.http://www.aosw.org/aosw/Main/About-AOSW/Mission-and-Goals/AOSWMain/About-AOSW/mission-and-goals.aspx?hkey=782e2be0-de81-4c24-af6d-36c11e7bca43.

"ASCO Profile and Mission Statement." American Society of Clinical Oncology. 2015. http://www.asco.org/about-asco/asco-profile-and-mission-statement.

Associated Press. "F.D.A. Clears Cancer Test That Uses Patients' DNA." *New York Times*, August 11, 2014. http://www.nytimes.com/2014/08/12/business/fda-clears-cancer-test-that-uses-patients-dna.html.

Balogh, Erin P., Patricia A. Ganz, Sharon B. Murphy, Sharyl J. Nass, Betty R. Ferrell, and Ellen Stovall. "Patient-Centered Cancer Treatment Planning: Improving the Quality of Oncology Care. Summary of an Institute of Medicine Workshop." *The Oncologist* 16 (2011): 1800–05. https://theoncologist.alphamedpress.org/content/16/12/1800.full.pdf.

Beishon, Marc. "A Second Opinion, Because There's No Second Chance." *Cancer World* (January/February 2007): 14–19. http://www.cancerworld.org/pdf/8775_CW16_14-19_GrandroundOK.pdf.

Berger, Ann M., Lynn H. Gerber, and Deborah K. Mayer. "Cancer-Related Fatigue." *Journal of National Comprehensive Cancer Network* 8, no. 8 (August 1, 2010): 904–31. http://www.jnccn.org/content/8/8/904.short.

"Biggest Cause of Personal Bankruptcy: Medical Bills." Today. June 25, 2013. http://www.today.com/money/biggest-cause-personal-bankruptcy-medical-bills-6C10442408.

Boyes, Allison W., Afaf Girgis, Catherine D'Este, and Alison C. Zucca. "Flourishing or Floundering? Prevalence and Correlates of Anxiety and Depression among a Population-Based Sample of Adult Cancer Survivors 6 Months after Diagnosis." *Journal of Affective Disorders* 135, nos. 1–3 (December 2011): 184–92. http://www.ncbi.nlm.nih.gov/pubmed/21864913.

Brett, Regina. "Regina Brett Quotes." Brainy Quote. http://www.brainyquote.com/quotes/quotes/r/reginabret586752.html.

Brintzenhofe-Szoc, Karlynn M., Tomer T. Levin, Yuelin Li, David W. Kissane, and James R. Zabora. "Mixed Anxiety/Depression Symptoms in a Large Cancer Cohort: Prevalence by Cancer Type." *Psychosomatics* 50, no. 4 (July–August 2009): 383–91. http://www.sciencedirect.com/science/article/pii/S0033318209708230.

Brody, Jane E. "When Treating Cancer Is Not an Option." *New York Times*, November 19, 2012. http://well.blogs.nytimes.com/2012/11/19/when-treating-cancer-is-not-an-option/?_php=true&_type=blogs&_r=0.

"Cancer and CAM: What the Science Says." *NCCAM Clinical Digest* (October 2010).

"Cancer Experience Registry." Cancer Support Community. 2014. https://csc.cancerexperienceregistry.org/.

Cancer Hope Network. http://www.cancerhopenetwork.org/.

Cancer.net. 2015. http://www.cancer.net/.

"Cancer Pain." Stanford Health Care. 2015. https://stanfordhealthcare.org/medical-conditions/pain/cancer-pain.html.

"Cancer Staging." National Cancer Institute. May 3, 2013. http://www.cancer.gov/cancertopics/factsheet/detection/staging.

"Cancer Symptoms, Signs and Prevention." CancerSymptoms.org. 2013. http://www.cancersymptoms.org/.

Casellas-Grau, Anna, Antoni Font, and Jaume Vives. "Positive Psychology Interventions in Breast Cancer: A Systematic Review." *Psycho-Oncology* 23, no. 1 (2014): 9–19. http://onlinelibrary.wiley.com/doi/10.1002/pon.3353/pdf.

Coalition of Cancer Cooperative Groups. 2013. http://www.cancertrialshelp.org/default.aspx.

Colosia, Ann D., Gerson Peltz, Gerhardt Pohl, Esther Liu, Kati Copley-Merriman, Shahnaz Khan, and James A. Kaye, "A Review and Characterization of the Various Perceptions of Quality Cancer Care." *Cancer* (March 1, 2011): 884–96. http://www.ncbi.nlm.nih.gov/pmc/articles/PMC3073118/pdf/cncr0117-0884.pdf.

Cowens-Alvarado, Rebecca, Katherine Sharpe, Mandi Pratt-Chapman, Anne Willis, Ted Gansler, Patricia A. Ganz, Stephen B. Edge, Mary S. McCabe, and Kevin Stein. "Advancing Survivorship Care through the National Cancer Survivorship Resource Center: Developing American Cancer Society Guidelines for Primary Care Providers." *CA: A Cancer Journal for Clinicians* 63, no. 3 (May/June 2013): 147–50. http://onlinelibrary.wiley.com/doi/10.3322/caac.21183/pdf.

"Distress in People with Cancer." American Cancer Society. Last modified August 13, 2014. http://www.cancer.org/acs/groups/cid/documents/webcontent/002827-pdf.pdf.

Documet, Patricia I., Jeanette M. Trauth, Meghan Key, Jason Flatt, and Jan Jernigan. "Breast Cancer Survivors' Perception of Survivorship." *Oncology Nursing Forum* 39, no. 3 (May 1, 2012): 309–15. http://www.ncbi.nlm.nih.gov/pmc/articles/PMC3437916/pdf/nihms398533.pdf.

Edwards, Elizabeth. "Elizabeth Edwards Quotes." BrainyQuote. http://www.brainyquote.com/quotes/authors/e/elizabeth_edwards.html.

Emanuel, Linda, Frank D. Ferris, Charles F. von Gunten, and Jaime H. Von Roenn, "Clarifying Diagnosis and Prognosis in Cancer: Guidance for Healthcare Providers." *Medscape* (March 30, 2011). http://www.medscape.org/viewarticle/739252.

"End-of-Life Care for People Who Have Cancer." National Cancer Institute. Last modified May 10, 2012. http://www.cancer.gov/cancertopics/factsheet/Support/end-of-life-care.

Ernst, Edzard. "Alternative Treatments for Breast Cancer." *European Journal of Clinical Pharmacology* 68 (2012): 434–54. http://paperity.org/p/19734319/alternative-treatments-for-breast-cancer.

Etheridge, Melissa. "Melissa Etheridge Quotes." BrainyQuote. http://www.brainyquote.com/quotes/authors/m/melissa_etheridge_2.html.

"The FDA's Drug Review Process: Ensuring Drugs Are Safe and Effective." U.S. Food and Drug Administration. Last modified November 6, 2014. http://www.fda.gov/drugs/resourcesforyou/consumers/ucm143534.htm.

Feiler, Bruce. "Cancer Survivors Celebrate Their Cancerversary." *New York Times*, December 8, 2013. http://www.nytimes.com/2013/12/08/fashion/Cancer-Survivors-five-year-Celebration-Day-known-as-cancerversary.html?_r=0.

"Food for Life: Cancer Project." Physicians Committee for Responsible Medicine. http://pcrm.org/health/cancer-resources.

Fujimori, Maiko, and Yosuke Uchitomi, "Preferences of Cancer Patients Regarding Communication of Bad News: A Systematic Literature Review." *Japan Journal of Clinical Oncology* 39, no. 4 (February 3, 2009): 201–16. http://jjco.oxfordjournals.org/content/39/4/201.full.pdf.

Furber, L., K. Cox, R. Murphy, and W. Steward, "Investigating Communication in Cancer Consultations: What Can Be Learned from Doctor and Patient Accounts of their Experience?" *European Journal of Cancer Care* 22 (2013): 653–62.

"Genetic Testing: What You Need to Know." American Cancer Society. Last modified October 18, 2013. http://www.cancer.org/cancer/cancercauses/geneticsandcancer/genetictesting/genetic-testing-who-should-test.

Gladwell, Malcolm. *Outliers*. New York: Little, Brown, 2008.

Glare, Paul. "Clinical Predictors of Survival in Advanced Cancer." *Journal of Supportive Oncology* 3, no. 5 (2005): 331–39.

Gorski, David. "Another Cancer Tragedy in the Making." Science-Based Medicine. May 14, 2012. http://www.sciencebasedmedicine.org/another-cancer-tragedy-in-the-making/.

Grunfeld, Eva, and Craig C. Earle. "The Interface between Primary and Oncology Specialty Care: Treatment through Survivorship." *Journal of the National Cancer Institute Monographs* 40 (2010): 25–30. http://jncimonographs.oxfordjournals.org/content/2010/40/25.full.pdf+html.

Gubar, Susan. "Living with Cancer: A Tour of Hospice." *New York Times,* July 24, 2014. http://well.blogs.nytimes.com/2014/07/24/living-with-cancer-a-tour-of-hospice/.

————. "Living with Cancer: Chronic, Not Cured," *New York Times,* June 5, 2014. http://well.blogs.nytimes.com/2014/06/05/living-with-cancer-chronic-not-cured/?_r=0.

————. "Living with Cancer: The New Medicine." *New York Times,* June 26, 2014. http://well.blogs.nytimes.com/2014/06/26/living-with-cancer-the-new-medicine/.

"Guidelines Urge Exercise for Cancer Patients, Survivors." *National Cancer Institute (NCI) Cancer Bulletin* 7, no. 3 (June 29, 2010).

Hagerty, Rebecca G., Phyllis N. Butow, Peter M. Ellis, Elizabeth A. Lobb, Susan C. Pendlebury, Natasha Leighl, Craig MacLeod, and Martin H. N. Tattersall. "Communicating with Realism and Hope: Incurable Cancer Patients' Views on the Disclosure of Prognosis." *Journal of Clinical Oncology* 23, no. 6 (February 20, 2005): 1278–88. http://jco.ascopubs.org/content/23/6/1278.full.pdf.

Hickey, Sonja Sherry. "Enabling Hope." *Cancer Nursing* 9, no. 3 (1986): 133–37.

Hinz, A., O. Krauss, J. P. Hauss, M. Jockel, R. D. Kortmann, J. U. Stolzenburg, and R. Schwarz. "Anxiety and Depression in Cancer Patients Compared with the General Population." *European Journal of Cancer Care* 19, no. 4 (July 2010): 522–29. http://onlinelibrary.wiley.com/doi/10.1111/j.1365-2354.2009.01088.x/abstract?systemMessage=Wiley+Online+Library+will+be+disrupted+Saturday%2C+15+March+from+10%3A00-12%3A00+GMT+%2806%3A00-08%3A00+EDT%29+for+essential+maintenance.

"History of Hospice Care." National Hospice and Palliative Care Organization. http://www.nhpco.org/history-hospice-care.

Horneber, Markus, Irene Fischer, Fernando Dimeo, Jens Ulrich Rüffer, and Joachim Weis. "Cancer-Related Fatigue: Epidemiology, Pathogenesis, Diagnosis, and Treatment." *Deutsches Arzteblatt International* 109, no. 9 (2012): 161–72. http://www.aerzteblatt.de/int/archive/article/122875/Cancer-Related-Fatigue-Epidemiology-Pathogenesis-Diagnosis-and-Treatment.

"Hospice Care." National Cancer Institute. Last modified October 25, 2012. http://www.cancer.gov/cancertopics/factsheet/Support/hospice.

"How to Find a Doctor or Treatment Facility If You Have Cancer." National Cancer Institute. Last modified June 5, 2013. http://www.cancer.gov/cancertopics/factsheet/Therapy/doctor-facility.

Jarvis, William T. "Cancer Quackery." National Council against Health Fraud. Last modified December 17, 2000. http://www.ncahf.org/articles/c-d/caquackery.html.

Jauhar, Sandeep. "When Doctors Need to Lie." *New York Times,* February 22, 2014. http://www.nytimes.com/2014/02/23/opinion/sunday/when-doctors-need-to-lie.html?_r=0.

Jenkins, Valerie, Ivonne Solis-Trapala, Carolyn Langridge, Susan Catt, Denis C. Talbot, and Leslie J. Fallowfield. "What Oncologists Believe They Said and What Patients Believe They Heard: An Analysis of Phase I Trial Discussions." *Journal of Clinical Oncology* 29, no. 1 (January 1, 2011): 61–68. http://jco.ascopubs.org/content/29/1/61.full.pdf.

Johnson, Kjel, Lee Blansett, Radha Mawrie, and Stefano Di Biase. *Innovation in Cancer Care and Implications for Health Systems: Global Oncology Trend Report.* Plymouth Meeting, PA: IMS Institute for Healthcare Informatics, 2014. http://www.imshealth.com/portal/site/imshealth/menuitem.762a961826aad98f53c753c71ad8c22a/?vgnextoid=f8d4df7a5e8b5410VgnVCM10000076192ca2RCRD.

Kantarjian, Hagop. "The Price of Drugs for Chronic Myeloid Leukemia (CML); A Reflection of the Unsustainable Prices of Cancer Drugs: From the Perspective of a Large Group of CML Experts." *Blood* (April 25, 2013). http://bloodjournal.hematologylibrary.org/content/early/2013/04/23/blood-2013-03-490003.full.pdf.

Katz, Steven J., and Monica Morrow. "Contralateral Prophylactic Mastectomy for Breast Cancer: Addressing Peace of Mind." *The Journal of the American Medical Association*

310, no. 8 (August 28, 2013): 793–94. http://jama.jamanetwork.com/article.aspx?articleid=1723134.

Keating, Nancy L., Mary Beth Landrum, Neeraj K. Arora, Jennifer L. Malin, Patricia A. Ganz, Michelle van Ryn, and Jane C. Weeks. "Cancer Patients' Role in Clinical Decisions: Do Characteristics of the Decision Influence Roles?" *Journal of Clinical Oncology* 28, no. 28 (October 1, 2010): 4364–70. http://jco.ascopubs.org/content/early/2010/08/16/JCO.2009.26.8870.full.pdf.

Khan, Nada F., Peter W. Rose, and Julie Evans. "Defining Cancer Survivorship: A More Transparent Approach Is Needed." *Journal of Cancer Survivorship* 6, no. 33 (2012): 33–36. http://link.springer.com/article/10.1007%2Fs11764-011-0194-6.

Klabunde, Carrie N., Paul K. J. Han, Craig C. Earle, Tenbroeck Smith, John Z. Ayanian, Richard Lee, Anita Ambs, Julia H. Rowland, and Arnold Potosky. "Physician Roles in the Cancer-Related Follow-Up Care of Cancer Survivors." *Family Medicine* 45, no. 7 (2013): 463–74. http://europepmc.org/articles/PMC3755767?pdf=render.

Kübler-Ross, Elisabeth. *On Death and Dying*. New York: Scribner, 1969.

Landro, Laura. "To Treat the Cancer, Treat the Distress." *Wall Street Journal*, August 27, 2012. http://online.wsj.com/news/articles/SB10000872396390444914904577615291424503430.

Laronga, Christine. "Patient Information: Breast Cancer Guide to Diagnosis and Treatment (Beyond the Basics)." UpToDate. Last modified September 26, 2013. http://www.uptodate.com/contents/breast-cancer-guide-to-diagnosis-and-treatment-beyond-the-basics.

"Learn about Clinical Studies." ClinicalTrials.gov. Last modified August 2012. http://www.clinicaltrials.gov/ct2/about-studies/learn.

Leifer, John. *The Myths of Modern Medicine: The Alarming Truth about American Health Care*. Lanham, MD: Rowman and Littlefield, 2014.

Lennes, Inga T., Jennifer S. Temel, Christen Hoedt, Ashley Meilleur, and Elizabeth B. Lamont. "Predictors of Newly Diagnosed Cancer Patients' Understanding of the Goals of Their Care at Initiation of Chemotherapy." *Cancer* (February 1, 2013): 691–99. http://www.ncbi.nlm.nih.gov/pmc/articles/PMC3531571/.

Linden, Wolfgang, Andrea Vodermaier, Regina MacKenzie, and Duncan Greig, "Anxiety and Depression after Cancer Diagnosis: Prevalence Rates by Cancer Type, Gender, and Age." *Journal of Affective Disorders* 141, nos. 2–3 (December 10, 2012): 343–51. http://www.sciencedirect.com/science/article/pii/S0165032712002212.

"Lynch Syndrome." Genetics Home Reference. Last modified May 2013. http://ghr.nlm.nih.gov/condition/lynch-syndrome.

Mack, Jennifer W., and Thomas J. Smith, "Reasons Why Physicians Do Not Have Discussions about Poor Prognosis, Why It Matters, and What Can Be Improved." *Journal of Clinical Oncology* 30, no. 22 (August 1, 2012): 2715–17. http://jco.ascopubs.org/content/30/22/2715.full.

"Managing the Costs of Your Cancer Treatment." American Cancer Society. Last modified August 4, 2014. http://www.cancer.org/treatment/findingandpayingfortreatment/managinginsuranceissues/the-cost-of-cancer-treatment.

Mao, Jun James, Christina Shearer Palmer, Kaitlin Elizabeth Healy, Krupali Desai, and Jay Amsterdam. "Complementary and Alternative Medicine Use among Cancer Survivors: A Population-Based Study." *Journal of Cancer Survivorship* 5, no. 1 (March 2011): 8–17. http://www.ncbi.nlm.nih.gov/pmc/articles/PMC3564962/pdf/nihms-438873.pdf.

Mayo Clinic Staff. "Cancer Treatment Decisions: 5 Steps to Help You Decide." Mayo Clinic. May 4, 2013. http://www.mayoclinic.org/diseases-conditions/cancer/in-depth/cancer-treatment/art-20047350.

"Medicine: Cancer Quacks." *Time*, February 28, 1955. http://content.time.com/time/magazine/article/0,9171,861227,00.html.

Medscape. http://www.medscape.com/.

Mellace, Jennifer. "The Financial Burden of Cancer Care." *Social Work Today* 10, no. 2 (March/April 2010): 14. http://www.socialworktoday.com/archive/032210p14.shtml.

Merckaert, Isabelle, Yves Libert, Sophie Messin, Mina Milani, Jean-Louis Slachmuylder, and Danius Razavi. "Cancer Patients' Desire for Psychological Support: Prevalence and Implications for Screening Patients' Psychological Needs." *Psycho-Oncology* 19, no. 2 (February 2010): 141–49. http://onlinelibrary.wiley.com/doi/10.1002/pon.1568/pdf.

Miller, Gabriel, Barrie R. Cassileth, and Edzard Ernst. "Asking the Experts: Complementary and Alternative Medicine and Cancer." Medscape. September 2, 2014. http://www.medscape.com/viewarticle/830553.

Mills, Moyra A., and Kate Sullivan. "The Importance of Information Giving for Patients Newly Diagnosed with Cancer: A Review of the Literature." *Journal of Clinical Nursing*, no. 8 (1999): 631–42.

Minogue, Kylie. "Kylie Minogue Quotes." BrainyQuote. http://www.brainyquote.com/quotes/authors/k/kylie_minogue.html.

Mitchell, Alex J., Nick Meader, Evan Davies, Kerrie Clover, Gregory L. Carter, Matthew J. Loscalzo, Wolfgang Linden, Luigi Grassi, Christoffer Johansen, Linda E. Carlson, and James Zabora. "Meta-Analysis of Screening and Case Finding Tools for Depression in Cancer: Evidence Based Recommendations for Clinical Practice on Behalf of the Depression in Cancer Care Consensus Group." *Journal of Affective Disorders* 140, no. 2 (October 2012): 149–60. http://www.sciencedirect.com/science/article/pii/S0165032711008068.

Mock, Victoria, Mary Pickett, Mary E. Ropka, Esther Muscari Lin, Kerry J. Stewart, Verna A. Rhodes, Roxanne McDaniel, Patricia M. Grimm, Sharon Krumm, and Ruth McCorkle. "Fatigue and Quality of Life Outcomes of Exercise during Cancer Treatment." *Cancer Practice* 9, no. 3 (May/June 2001): 119–27.

Nadel, Jeffrey, and Kavita Patel. "Changing the Way We Pay for Cancer Care." Brookings Institute. June 9, 2014. http://www.brookings.edu/research/opinions/2014/06/09-cancer-care-payment-reform-patel.

Nagy, Rebecca, Kevin Sweet, and Charis Eng. "Highly Penetrant Hereditary Cancer Syndromes." *Oncogene* 23, no. 38 (2004): 6445–70. http://www.nature.com/onc/journal/v23/n38/full/1207714a.html.

"NCCIH Facts-at-a-Glance and Mission." National Center for Complementary and Integrative Health. Last modified January 9, 2015. https://nccih.nih.gov/about/ataglance.

"NCCS Mission." National Coalition for Cancer Survivorship. 2015. http://www.canceradvocacy.org/about-us/our-mission/.

"NCI Mission Statement." National Cancer Institute. http://www.cancer.gov/aboutnci/overview/mission.

"Nearly One Third of Medicare Patients with Advanced Cancer Die in Hospitals and ICUs; About Half Get Hospice Care." Dartmouth Institute for Health Policy and Clinical Practice. November 16, 2010. http://www.dartmouthatlas.org/downloads/press/Cancer_report_release_111610.pdf.

"NHPCO's Facts and Figures: Hospice Care in America." National Hospice and Palliative Care Organization. 2013. http://www.nhpco.org/sites/default/files/public/Statistics_Research/2013_Facts_Figures.pdf.

Northouse, Laurel L., Maria Katapodi, Lixin Song, Lingling Zhang, and Darlene W. Mood. "Interventions with Family Caregivers of Cancer Patients: Meta-Analysis of Randomized Trials." *CA: A Cancer Journal for Clinicians* 60, no. 5 (2010): 317–39. http://www.ncbi.nlm.nih.gov/pmc/articles/PMC2946584/pdf/nihms208009.pdf.

"Nutrition for the Person with Cancer during Treatment: A Guide for Patients and Families." American Cancer Society. Last modified June 9, 2014. http://www.cancer.org/acs/groups/cid/documents/webcontent/002903-pdf.pdf.

"Nutrition in Cancer Care (PDQ)." National Cancer Institute. Last modified December 5, 2014. http://www.cancer.gov/cancertopics/pdq/supportivecare/nutrition/Patient/page1/AllPages.

"Our History and Mission." Patient Advocate Foundation. 2012. http://www.patientadvocate.org/about.php?p=906.

"Pain Management—Pain Management." Community Health Network. n.d. http://www.ecommunity.com/health/index.aspx?pageID=P07302.

"Pain (PDQ)." National Cancer Institute. Last updated April 10, 2014. http://www.cancer. gov/cancertopics/pdq/supportivecare/pain/Patient/page1/AllPages.

"Palliative Care in Cancer." National Cancer Institute. Last modified March 16, 2010. http:// www.cancer.gov/cancertopics/factsheet/Support/palliative-care.

Parker-Pope, Tara. "Scientists Seek to Rein in Diagnoses of Cancer." *New York Times*, July 29, 2013. http://well.blogs.nytimes.com/2013/07/29/report-suggests-sweeping-changes-to-cancer-detection-and-treatment/?action=click&module=Search&region= searchResults%230&version=&url=http%3A%2F%2Fquery.nytimes.com%2Fse.

"Patient and Caregiver Resources." National Comprehensive Cancer Network. 2014. http:// www.nccn.org/patients/advocacy/default.aspx.

"Patient-Centered Sites." Association of Cancer Online Resources. 2015. http://www.acor. org/pages/resources.

Pausch, Randy. "Randy Pausch's Web Site." Carnegie Mellon University. http://www.cs.cmu. edu/~pausch/.

Peikoff, Kira. "Fearing Punishment for Bad Genes." *New York Times*, April 7, 2014. http:// www.nytimes.com/2014/04/08/science/fearing-punishment-for-bad-genes.html.

Pelzer, Dave. "Dave Pelzer Quotes." BrainyQuote. http://www.brainyquote.com/quotes/ authors/d/dave_pelzer.html.

Perlman, Adam, Oliver Lontok, Maureen Huhmann, J. Scott Parrott, Leigh Ann Simmons, and Linda Patrick-Miller. "Prevalence and Correlates of Postdiagnosis Initiation of Complementary and Alternative Medicine among Patients at a Comprehensive Cancer Center." *Journal of Oncology Practice* 9, no. 1 (January 2013): 34–41. http://www.ncbi.nlm. nih.gov/pmc/articles/PMC3545661/pdf/jop34.pdf.

Philip, Jennifer, Michelle Gold, Max Schwarz, and Paul Komesaroff. "Second Medical Opinions: The Views of Oncology Patients and Their Physicians." *Supportive Care in Cancer* 18, no. 9 (September 2010): 1199–1205. http://www.ncbi.nlm.nih.gov/pubmed/19802635.

Pollack, Andrew. "Doctors Denounce Cancer Drug Prices of $100,000 a Year." *New York Times*, April 25, 2013. http://www.nytimes.com/2013/04/26/business/cancer-physicians-attack-high-drug-costs.html.

———. "Drug Saves Fertility for Women with Cancer." *New York Times*, May 30, 2014. http://www.nytimes.com/2014/05/31/business/drug-could-protect-fertility-in-breast-cancer-patients.html.

Potosky, Arnold L., Paul K. J. Han, Julia Rowland, Carrie N. Klabunde, Tenbroeck Smith, Noreen Aziz, Craig Earle, John Z. Ayanian, Patricia A. Ganz, and Michael Stefanek. "Differences between Primary Care Physicians' and Oncologists' Knowledge, Attitudes and Practices Regarding the Care of Cancer Survivors." *Journal of General Internal Medicine* 26, no. 12 (December 2011): 1403–10. http://link.springer.com/article/10.1007/ s11606-011-1808-4#page-1.

Rabin, Roni Caryn. "In Israel, a Push to Screen for Cancer Gene Leaves Many Conflicted." *New York Times*, November 26, 2011. http://www.nytimes.com/2013/11/27/health/in-israel-a-push-to-screen-for-cancer-gene-leaves-many-conflicted.html.

Reb, Anne C. "Transforming the Death Sentence: Elements of Hope in Women with Advanced Ovarian Cancer." *Oncology Nursing Forum* 73, no. 6 (2007): 70–81.

Rieber, Alyssa G. "How Being a Cancer Survivor Affects My Oncology Practice." *ASCO Connection*, April 22, 2014. http://connection.asco.org/Magazine/Article/ID/3852/How-Being-a-Cancer-Survivor-Affects-My-Oncology-Practice.aspx.

"The Right Care at the Right Time: Hospice Length of Stay." Hospice Action Network. 2014. http://hospiceactionnetwork.org/linked_documents/get_informed/policy_resources/ PolicyBriefing_LengthofStay_March2014.pdf.

Riley, Bronson D., Julie O. Culver, Cecile Skrzynia, Leigha A. Senter, June A. Peters, Josephine W. Costalas, Faith Callif-Daley, Sherry C. Grumet, Katherine S. Hunt, Rebecca S. Nagy, Wendy C. McKinnon, Nancie M. Petrucelli, Robin L. Bennett, and Angela M. Trepanier. "Essential Elements of Genetic Cancer Risk Assessment, Counseling, and Testing: Updated Recommendations of the National Society of Genetic Counselors." *Journal of Genetic Counseling* 21 (2012): 151–61.

Roth, Bruce J., Lada Krilov, Sylvia Adams, Carol A. Aghajanian, Peter Bach, Fadi Braiteh, Marcia S. Brose, Lee M. Ellis, Harry Erba, Daniel J. George, Mark R. Gilbert, Joseph O. Jacobson, Eric C. Larsen, Stuart M. Lichtman, Ann H. Partridge, Jyoti D. Patel, David I. Quinn, Leslie L. Robison, Jamie H. von Roenn, Wolfram Samlowski, Gary K. Schwartz, and Nicholas J. Vogelzang. "Clinical Cancer Advances 2012: Annual Report on Progress against Cancer from the American Society of Clinical Oncology." *Journal of Clinical Oncology* 31, no. 1 (January 1, 2013): 131–61.

"Royal Rife." Wikipedia. http://en.wikipedia.org/wiki/Royal_Rife.

Russell, Bethany J., and Alicia M. Ward, "Deciding What Information Is Necessary: Do Patients with Advanced Cancer Want to Know All the Details?" *Cancer Management and Research* 3 (2011): 191–99.

Schaepe, Karen Sue. "Bad News and First Impressions: Patient and Family Caregiver Accounts of Learning the Cancer Diagnosis." *Social Science in Medicine* 73, no. 6 (September 2011): 912–21. http://www.sciencedirect.com/science/article/pii/S0277953611004060.

Schenker, Yael, Alicia Fernandez, Rebecca Sudore, and Dean Schillinger, "Interventions to Improve Patient Comprehension in Informed Consent for Medical and Surgical Procedures: A Systematic Review." *Medical Decision Making* 31, no. 1(January–February 2011): 151–73. http://mdm.sagepub.com/content/31/1/151.short.

Schmitz, Kathryn H., Kerry S. Courneya, Charles Matthews, Wendy Demark-Wahnefried, Daniel A. Galvao, Bernadine M. Pinto, Melinda L. Irwin, Kathleen Y. Wolin, Roanne J. Segal, Alejandro Lucia, Carole M. Schneider, Vivian E. von Gruenigen, and Anna L. Schwartz. "American College of Sports Medicine Roundtable on Exercise Guidelines for Cancer Survivors." *Medicine and Science in Sports and Exercise* 42, no. 7 (July 2010): 1409–26. https://www.penncancer.org/pdf/pal/American_College_of_Sports_Medicine_Roundtable_on_23.pdf.

"Search for Clinical Trials." National Cancer Institute. http://www.cancer.gov/clinicaltrials/search.

Sepkowitz, Kent A. "Looking for the Final Word on Treatment." *New York Times*, May 14, 2014.   http://www.nytimes.com/2014/05/14/health/looking-for-the-final-word-on-treatment.html?_r=0.

Siegel, Rebecca, Carol DeSantis, Katherin Virgo, Kevin Stein, Angela Mariotto, Tenbroeck Smith, Dexter Cooper, Ted Gansler, Catherine Lerro, Stacey Fedewa, Chunchieh Lin, Corinne Leach, Rachel Spillers Cannady, Hyunsoon Cho, Steve Scoppa, Mark Hachey, Rebecca Kirch, Ahmedin Jemal, and Elizabeth Ward. "Cancer Treatment and Survivorship Statistics." *CA: A Cancer Journal for Clinicians* 62, no. 4 (July/August 2012): 220–41. http://onlinelibrary.wiley.com/doi/10.3322/caac.21149/pdf.

Smith, Peter J., Alexandra Clavarino, Jeremy Long, and Kathryn J. Steadman. "Why Do Some Cancer Patients Receiving Chemotherapy Choose to Take Complementary and Alternative Medicines and What Are the Risks?" *Asia-Pacific Journal of Clinical Oncology* 10, no. 1 (March 2014): 1–10. http://onlinelibrary.wiley.com/doi/10.1111/ajco.12115/abstract;jsessionid=B9CC99FF876B420DF4063ADC14921E51.f04t02?systemMessage=Wiley+Online+Library+will+be+disrupted+Saturday%2C+15+March+from+10%3A00-12%3A00+GMT+%2806%3A00-08%3A00+EDT%29+for+essential+maintenance.

Smith, Thomas J., Lindsay A. Dow, Enid A. Virago, James Khatcheressian, Robin Matsuyama, and Laurel J. Lyckholm, "A Pilot Trial of Decision Aids to Give Truthful Prognostic and Treatment Information to Chemotherapy Patients with Advanced Cancer." *Journal of Supportive Oncology* 9, no. 2 (2011): 79–86. http://www.ncbi.nlm.nih.gov/pmc/articles/PMC3589716/pdf/nihms-447553.pdf.

"SOAPP (Symptom Outcomes and Practice Patterns)." Eastern Cooperative Oncology Group. 2012. http://www.ecogsoapp.com/about.html.

Span, Paula. "How to Choose a Hospice." *New York Times*, June 17, 2014. http://newoldage.blogs.nytimes.com/2014/06/17/how-to-choose-a-hospice/.

———. "When Advance Directives Are Ignored." *New York Times*, June 24, 2014. http://newoldage.blogs.nytimes.com/2014/06/24/when-advance-directives-are-ignored/.

Stenger, Matthew. "Nurse Navigators Improve Patient-Reported Quality of Care in Early Cancer Care." *ASCO Post*, December 3, 2013. http://www.ascopost.com/ViewNews.aspx?nid=10799.

Tarkan, Laurie. "Value of Second Opinions Is Underscored in Study of Biopsies." *The New York Times*, April 4, 2000. http://www.nytimes.com/2000/04/04/health/value-of-second-opinions-is-underscored-in-study-of-biopsies.html.

Thorne, Sally, T., Gregory Hislop, Charmaine Kim-Sing, Valerie Oglov, John L. Oliffe, and Kelly I. Stajduhar. "Changing Communication Needs and Preferences across the Cancer Care Trajectory: Insights from the Patient Perspective." *Supportive Care in Cancer* 22, no. 4 (April 2014): 1009–15. http://link.springer.com/article/10.1007/s00520-013-2056-4.

"Trim Your Cancer Risk with Exercise," Fred Hutchinson Cancer Research Center. 2015. https://www.fhcrc.org/en/events/healthy-living/Trim-Risk.html.

Underhill, Meghan L., and Cheryl B. Crotser. "Seeking Balance: Decision Support Needs of Women without Cancer and a Deleterious BRCA1 or BRCA2 Mutation." *Journal of Genetic Counseling* 23, no. 3 (November 22, 2013), 1–13.

Valdivieso, Manuel, Ann M. Kujawa, Tisha Jones, and Laurence H. Baker. "Cancer Survivors in the United States: A Review of the Literature and a Call to Action." *International Journal of Medical Sciences* 9, no. 2 (2012): 163–73. http://www.ncbi.nlm.nih.gov/pmc/articles/PMC3264952/pdf/ijmsv09p0163.pdf.

Weissman, David E. "Fast Fact #13: Determining Prognosis in Advanced Cancer." Center to Advance Palliative Care. Last modified March 2009. https://www.capc.org/fast-facts/13-determining-prognosis-advanced-cancer/.

"Welcome." Bone and Cancer Foundation. 2011. http://www.boneandcancerfoundation.org/.

Wennberg, John, and Alan Gittelsohn. "Small Area Variations in Health Care Delivery." *Science* 182, no. 4117 (December 1973): 1102–8. doi:10.1126/science.182.4117.1102.

"What We Do." Prevent Cancer Foundation. http://preventcancer.org/what-we-do/.

"What You Need to Know as a Cancer Caregiver." American Cancer Society. Last modified April 28, 2014. http://www.cancer.org/acs/groups/cid/documents/webcontent/acspc-027595-pdf.pdf.

"Where the Money Goes." LiveStrong Foundation. http://www.livestrong.org/what-we-do/our-approach/where-the-money-goes/.

Woelk, Cornelius J. "How Long Have I Got?" *Canadian Family Physician* 55 (December 2009): 1202–6.

Zafar, S. Yousuf. "How Should We Assess and Address the Financial Toxicity of Cancer Care?" *ASCO Connection*, April 22, 2014. http://connection.asco.org/Magazine/Article/ID/3849/Cost-of-Cancer-Care-A-Crucial-Physician-Patient-Conversation.aspx.

INDEX